SWAN BOOKS

To/ Denny Walters

May the energy

in you and me

be happily used

thru this book,

6/19/02

George Wishlin, M.D.

GEORGE NICKLIN, M.D.
DOCTORS IN PERIL
HOW THEY COPE

First Printing June 2000
1
Designed, Printed & Manufactured by M.B.G.& A., Inc.
735 Calebs Path, Glaro Bldg., Hauppauge, NY 11788

Cover Design by Jim Vincent/MBG&A, Inc.

Published by Swan Books, Main Street, Pine Plains, NY 12567
©2000 Geroge Nicklin, M.D., all rights reserved

Library of Congress Catalog Card Number: 00-90221
International Standard Book Number: 0-940429-23-3

For information, please address: George Nicklin, M.D.,
6 Butler Place, Garden City, NY 11530

Editor and Author
GEORGE NICKLIN, M.D.
Associate Clinical Professor
New York University School of Medicine

Introduction written by
ROBERT CANCRO, M.D., M.ed.,D.Sc.
Professor and Chairman of Psychiatry
New York University School of Medicine

DOCTORS IN PERIL
How They Cope

Published by

SWAN BOOKS
Main Street
Pine Plains, NY 12567

Designed, Printed & Manufactured in the U.S.A. by

MBG&A
Hauppauge, New York 11788

Dedicated to my wife
Kate Aronson Nicklin

ACKNOWLEDGMENTS

I would like to express my gratitude for the help that I received from many people but primarily from my secretaries Nancy Meegan, Erica Rechsteiner, Lillian Landsberger, Carolyn Bertrand, Jodi Pearlman and Virginia Curley.

I am especially indebted to Robert Cancro M.D, my department head at New York University's Department of Psychiatry. He both encouraged and assisted me in realizing publication of this book and in writing its introduction.

The most significant person, who I feel in a way was heaven sent, is my most recent personal assistant Maureen K. Lane, who arrived a year ago and has been a wonderful worker on this document. She edited the book, addressing both its style and its coherence, thereby speeding its conclusion. While I feel that all of my coworkers have been heaven sent, this is certainly most clear with Maureen K. Lane.

TABLE OF CONTENTS

PREFACE

"Sweet are the uses of adversity;
Which, like the toad, ugly and venomous,
Wears yet a precious jewel in his head."

Shakespeare (As You Like It Act II, Sc. 1)

What is the purpose of this book? The purpose is to give both the laity and other physicians an opportunity to see how doctors at peril either cope successfully with severe medical conditions or else fail and succumb to their conditions. Its purpose is also to prolong and enhance the lives of others.

Physicians are informed consumers of health services and as such should be able to obtain the best services available. It is therefore of use to us to see how well they in fact cope when faced with life threatening problems.

Some 55 years ago, at the tender age of 19, I found myself locked in mortal combat. During the years 1944-45, it was usual for a white male American of my age group to be propelled somewhere into the heart of combat in the battles of World War II. My experience was no different from that of hundreds of thousands of combatants on either side of the conflict struggling for a different set of ideals.

Looking back I see how these high ideals sustained me as I remained month after month and battle after battle on the front-lines of the war. We were winning but I knew that inevitably the odds would catch up with me as they had with most of my comrades-in-arms. For the first eight weeks I had been a rifleman and a mortar gunner "dogface", the man "who must win the war", fighting at the edge of our social order to extend it. A mortar gunner has more enhanced killing ability. At the end of the first two months I realized my unit of 100 - 120 men had been replaced about two and a half times. I observed comrades go mad, be wounded and die as I, seemingly fortunate, fought on.

Before the war I had wanted to become a physician but that plan was disrupted by the war after an introductory premedical term. But once in the army, I was more attentive to my personal medical care (from chiggers to lice to colds to athletes foot) than the regular soldier. I had treatments that were usually effective for these disorders e.g. sulfur tablets for "chiggers" (mites that cause severe itching), 24 hour hydrotherapy (much drinking of water - still incorporated into my practice) for respiratory infections, DDT ("dichlorodiphenyl-trichoroethane") for lice, foot powder for athletes foot and dry socks plus foot massage twice daily for the prevention of trench foot. I found myself being regularly consulted by my fellow soldiers as to how to deal with these medical disorders for which I had found effective therapies.

Our medics ran the highest casualty rates in combat and we were always short two or three of the four medics required in our company men. Soon I found myself being forced by superior officers to be a medic replacement. After a short introductory first aid course, I spent my remaining ten weeks on the front as a medic. This was during the time of the Battle of the Bulge (Dec. 16, 1944 - Jan. 16, 1945) and the Battle for Germany (Jan. 17, 1945 - Feb. 19, 1945).

From the beginning of the United States' involvement in World War II, Secretary of War, Henry Stimson, wanted to have a highly intelligent elite group of soldiers who would be ready to be introduced into the final battles of the war. He established these elite units in the Army and the Navy, giving them special titles. The Navy programs were called V-12 and V-5 (V for victory). The equivalent Army program was the Army's Specialized Training Program. The minimum IQ requirement for these programs, based on an admission screening test for the Armed Services, had to be 115. It is a reflection of the calibre of the physicians contributing to this book that six out of the twelve were members of the Army's Specialized Training Program. Five of these six received their medical training through the program. One of the six, admitted into the program at a later date, was sent directly to the infantry and completed his medical training after the war.

This book is a collection of contributions from physicians who were involved in war, who have suffered from typhus and tuberculosis - who have sustained massive physical injuries requiring lengthy hospitalization - and who have been in concentration camps. While only three of the physicians write directly about their war experiences, all but one of the others have been exposed to war.

Our wartime experiences were much as depicted in the movie "Saving Private Ryan". But on the far side of adversity can lie incredible opportunity and this was true of my life as well as that of others who survived. Many, of course, did not. 50,000 U.S. soldiers lost their lives in the Battle of the Bulge, and many more were wounded physically or emotionally in ways which impair them to this day. But those whose wounds and psyches did heal, myself included, have moved forward in their civilian lives and careers. The adversity which the war inflicted on us has became a tremendous asset. I have used it to discover new ways to survive effectively and to help others. I have become optimistic about life.

As I met other physicians with similar experiences to mine, I found their stories useful and also exciting. Three of the doctors in our collection have since died from their illnesses. But the stories of how they fought until the end and how this struggle had a positive effect on others provides valuable insight and hope for others.

The last to die was the victim of an atypically long, twelve year bout with Lou Gehrig's Disease ("Amyotrophic Lateral Sclerosis", "ALS"). He was severely disabled and had been so for many years. It is extremely worthwhile to see how he conquered the physical deterioration, stayed alive, and maintained his positive mental attitude for such an extended period of time.

The remaining physicians are in good health at the time of this writing. There is one who has coped successfully with cancer. Another has had to deal with the constant presence of death facing himself and very close members of his family. He has also had to deal with deafness which he considers a minor problem. Yet another found himself on the wrong side of a medical experiment and another had his health seriously compromised by some of the physicians whom he had selected to treat him.

In sharing all these experiences we hope to aid others and to provide hope as you move forward into the future. We all hope that our contributions to this work will benefit you in your ability to cope with your own medical problems. We hope that this will extend your life expectancy and that it will enable you to have a healthier, happier and more successful life.

Editor, George Nicklin, M.D.

INTRODUCTION

Life in all its various forms is a highly improbable occurrence. The natural state of the material universe is disorga-
nized resulting in powerful entropic forces which lead to decay.
Yet life exists and persists. This raises a number of philosophical
and perhaps even theological questions, which are beyond
the scope of this volume. This volume recognizes that all humans must confront adversity in all its multiple forms. The
confrontation can lead to collapse or to efforts to cope with
adversity. Not all coping efforts are equally successful in delay-
ing entropy and sustaining the organism in a satisfactory state
of equilibrium.

While adversity has many faces, there are several that all
humans will come to know. For humans, severe stress, illness
and death are absolute certainties. At different points in our
lives, we deal with them with different mechanisms. As children and as young adults death is usually an unreal abstrac-
tion. In late life it is often a compelling presence. Virtually all
humans recognize that illness and death are inevitable, therefore differences in how they deal with them become an important issue. Human beings will cope with these eventuali-

ties in very different ways, some of which are more adaptive than others. Because doctors devote their professional lives to working with illness and death they may well have some better understanding than individuals who have less extensive exposure and experience. This is not to suggest that doctors have superior intellects or coping skills, but rather that experience can be the best teacher and doctors may learn from watching how others manage in the face of their adversities.

The editor of this book believes that many people can benefit from the experiences of doctors who have had to face serious health risks ranging from cardiac to combat. This is a particularly important consideration as data begins to emerge suggesting that coping strategies can prolong life even in a fatal illness. A recent study demonstrated that women with metastatic breast cancer, who were in support groups, lived longer than matched controls who did not obtain the emotional support of the groups. As indicated earlier, life is a highly improbable fact. It is also a fact which we understand only minimally. The transition from life to death is inevitable, but the process may well be open to influences that go beyond medication and surgery. Variables such as a positive outlook, firm family support, strong friendship patterns and a continued commitment to life's activities can make a difference in both quality and duration of life.

The authors of these chapters are not professional writers. That is both an asset and a liability. The lack of "professionalism" brings a sincerity and an immediacy to the writing. Each chapter differs in style and in content.

They are not written with a single voice. Some experiences may offer little to a particular reader, while others may have a profound impact. The quality of the writing is not always "professional" but it is always "real". The unevenness in writing in my judgment is on balance an asset. Each chapter reflects life's frustrations and failures as well as successes. The book captures the fact that life is not a well manicured lawn, but rather a natural wilderness. In that wilderness there are treasures and dangers.

It is pointless in my opinion to summarize one or more chapters. There are messages to be heard and some to be rejected by the <u>individual</u> reader. While these are true "stories", they are much more than that. They represent an educational effort through baring and sharing of painful experiences. Unlike some popular television shows, they do not deal with the bizarre but rather the commonplace challenges faced by humans.

The chapters also reflect differences in individual ways of coping with the problems being faced. Some readers will relate more to the specific problem, while others will be more responsive to the coping strategies utilized. Ultimately, the message of the various writers is that frightening and noxious events can have a powerful positive transforming effect on the individual. Adversity can in fact strengthen a person's character. This is an important lesson that became diminished and almost lost during the culture wars of the 1960's. Individuals must struggle and can benefit from that struggle. Growth emerges from being tested and being forced to find where in fact our limits are, rather than where we thought they were. In that sense, this is a book of hope rather than of despair. That is not to say that one may not sense the anger that goes with fear and disappointment, but what is of greater importance is the triumph over these negative feelings and the gratitude and balance that can so frequently emerge.

Robert Cancro, M.D.
Lucius N. Littauer Professor of Psychiatry
Chairman of the Department of Psychiatry
Medical School
New York University
June 1999

DOCTORS IN PERIL

How They Cope

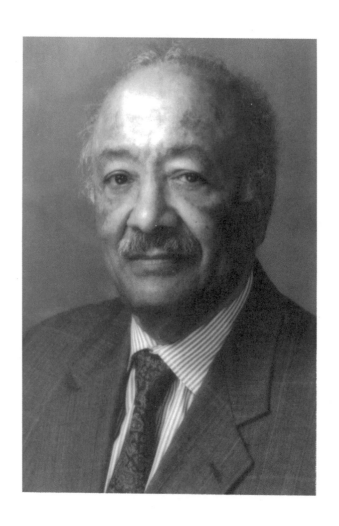

Earl L. Biassey, M.D.

MULTIPLE SYSTEMS FAILURE

Earle L. Biassey, M.D.

I remember only too well when I was in analysis and my analyst became ill. My early anxiety increased as speculation followed. All I knew was that my analyst was not available. I was relieved to finally discover that she was suffering from exhaustion and not from a severe heart attack. When I was asked to write this paper and share my feelings, I first thought in terms of my patients and their responses to my illness.

What does a doctor, particularly a psychoanalyst, do when he becomes the patient? He must consider his family, his patients and himself. How does he address his responsibilities? What priority does he give to them?

It is all a matter of transference. This is what he is trained to deal with. If the analyst is careless about his own health, his use to others is seriously undermined. When I first went into clinical practice I remarked to a considerably older colleague that I was extremely busy. His response was: "You're of use to no one if you're six feet under." Imposing perspective on one's priorities can be a source of conflict. Like children, analysts can unconsciously view themselves as invincible, immune to the negative vagaries of life.

My hypertension was first diagnosed in 1965 during a routine physical examination. It was controlled by medication for over 20 years. In the summer of 1989 I noticed swelling of my ankles. I attributed this to bilateral varicosities. Support stockings were prescribed by my physician and I considered the problem resolved. During the fall tennis season, I became so winded while playing that I stopped playing and left the court. I knew of no reason for this shortness of breath. Concurrently I was being treated for a prolonged bout of the flu, an illness that seemed to exist interminably. My electrocardiograms and chest x-rays had been normal yet the flu symptoms persisted. I suffered from a chronic cough.

For the first time in many years of practice, I found myself incapable of going to the office and of functioning effectively. At night my only comfort was to sit rather than lie down. I ignored this fact and others. I did not use my clinical acumen as an internist to diagnose symptoms that would have been evident to me in another individual. I failed to notice very clear warning signs. My denial continued for an extended period. The denial was co-opted by my colleagues and sanctioned by my desire to pursue my diversified interests: tennis, music, collections, patients and family.

In November 1989, my internist suggested that I see a pulmonary specialist. I spent a long afternoon in the specialist's office. He repeated chest x-rays and EKG's. After considerable review of the data, he indicated that I should be hospitalized - that night. My cardiac rhythm was highly irregular, proceeding at a galloping pace. I was in total congestive heart failure due to hypertension. I was placed on a ward with monitors, given intravenous medication and spent the next two weeks in the cardiac unit. I lost 60 pounds, mostly fluid, during this period.

During the first two days of hospitalization, I was unable to void and spent an agonizing night. I was finally catheterized and over 1,000 cc's of urine were taken from me. A consulting urologist said in a casual, almost blasé fashion, "You have hypertrophy. No real problem." However, as soon as the Foley Catheter was removed, I again obstructed.

The next element of my medical sequence was a "Roto Rooter Operation", a boring through of the urethra aperture. The next morning I was advised by my urologist: "Well, you have a few cancer cells." A medical decision was made that I should undergo radiation therapy. Surgery was perceived as too life-threatening. For the next six weeks as an outpatient, I underwent radiation therapy. The dosage of radiation was closely calibrated and the prostate was approached in a circular fashion a little bit at a time. There were minimal side effects and I felt well throughout the six weeks. Fortunately the hospital is only ten minutes from my office. I underwent this treatment while maintaining my usual office procedures and appointments.

I've continued to be treated by my cardiologist with high doses of medication. Alcohol is toxic to my body so

I totally abstain from alcohol consumption. My diet was a salt-free one. I was placed on anti-tensive medication, first Capote and a Catapres Patch. Dynacerc, a calcium blocker, effectively addressed my high blood pressure. The irregular rhythm was managed with fairly high doses of Quinaglut to which Mexitil is added. The arrhythmia was gradually brought under control. I was also prescribed a small amount of Lanoxin, a diuretic called Lasix and a potassium replacement, k-tabs.

Several months after the radiation treatment, I began to have a relentless hematuria. The hematuria was complicated by clotting resultant in frequent periods of obstruction. This caused considerable pain necessitating frequent trips to the emergency room or to the urology service. On numerous occasions I left home for the office, suffered pain from the obstruction, and had to return to the emergency room.

To control the bleeding, I was given Amicar, amino ceproic acid. It is an effective inhibitor of fibrinolysis. Urinary fibrinolysis is usually a normal physiological phenomenon associated with life-threatening complications subsequent to anoxia and severe shock symptomatic of such complications as surgical hematuria following prostatectomy and trans-uretheral resection ("TUR"). Because the bleeding persisted, a TUR was ultimately performed. Throughout this period, I continued to go to my office. My family and patients eventually persuaded me to remain at home. I was advised not to ride in a car even as a passenger.

The bleeding continued. My urologist informed me that I was losing so much blood that a transfusion would probably be necessary. The complications that would result from using my children's blood rather than the hospital's made me very wary of transfusions. My urologist also considered treating me with a strong hormone that would be uncomfortable and expensive, but perhaps necessary. Lastly he spoke of the possibility of an orchidectomy. Miraculously, it was three days after the latter proposal that the bleeding stopped.

Throughout this time I maintained contact with my most critical patients by telephone. They tried their best not to be overly troublesome. Several patients indicated their concern about my health. (One of these patients' concerns provides an addendum to this paper.) That is a summation of the contact and feelings that are of a transferential nature with my patients.

A further complication developed to exacerbate the preexisting ones. I began to have direct rectal bleeding with clots. I went to see another doctor, a proctologist, who made a diagnosis of radiation colonitis. He indicated that the radiation had caused the small capillaries to become very fragile causing bleeding to occur periodically from that end of the colon. I began a period of monitoring through colonostomy. The bleeding persisted though the source of the bleeding had been ascertained. A more thorough examination occurred next. Instead of going up two and a half feet, the doctor went up four feet to check for polyps in both the ascending and descending colon. He found several polyps in the lower descending colon which he removed. These were benign. I continue to be monitored.

Three years have passed since my original hospitalization. My cardiologist is pleased with my progress but he continues to monitor me. I have had to restrict my exercising. Most cardiological problems can be mitigated through exercise. In my case the obverse was true. Last Christmas my wife gave me an Alpine exerciser. My cardiologist hit the roof. He explained that 5% of people with cardiac problems are severely restricted as to exercise. He didn't even want me to walk up a hill on a cold winter day without shielding my air intake. Without taking this precaution, this type of walking could induce stress. I listened and acted accordingly but with extreme reluctance.

I continue to be monitored by my urologist and radiologist. The enzyme studies are normal. Every six months I'm alternately seen by the urologist and by the radiologist.

When I'm queried as to retirement, I respond, "An analyst never retires, he just loses his patience." I would be lost without some natural professional stimulation. I realize, however, that my life is not exclusively dependent upon work to provide its momentum. I now have grandchildren and diversified interests to enhance the quality of my life. Several years ago, I returned to singing and formal voice lessons. I later joined the chancellor choir at church and now sing every week at services. Each Christmas I sing in the concert series consisting of seven performances, I began to play the guitar and more recently to study piano. I continue to enjoy water color painting, sculpting and stamp collecting.

What have I learned and what can I share? When I reflect upon my life and the quality of that life, I have concluded that I do not have absolute control over many things. I am not omnipotent nor am I omniscient. I can exert a positive influence, cognizant of the brevity of life and the importance of relationships. I can do everything in my power to prevent all but the inevitable.

We must choose our doctors wisely, trust them and follow their orders assiduously. We should be completely candid with our physicians and give them the information that is critical to the resolution of our medical problems. My inspiration concerning medical knowledge is inspired by the wisdom of Sirach, who wrote in Ecclesiasticus 38:1-2: "Value the service of a doctor, for he has a place assigned him by The Lord. His skill comes from the Most High and he is rewarded by kings."

In conclusion, the following is a vignette written by one of my patients. I think it sums up the essence of patient care as far as a psychoanalyst is concerned.

My Biggest Fear

A lot of people might think that my biggest fear would be being told I was HIV positive. While that is frightening, it is not my biggest fear. My biggest fear is losing my psychiatrist or for that matter anyone I love. Dr. Biassey told me that at his next convention, one of the topics to be discussed was the therapist's illness and how doctor and patient deal with this. Both Dr. Biassey and I have dealt with this issue. In 1989, Dr. B. ended up in the hospital with a heart problem. Later he was told he had prostate cancer. When his heart problem was stabilized, he had radiation treatments and then had his prostate removed. This operation was followed by some problems.

I don't know whether it is considered okay for a patient to visit her hospitalized doctor, but Dr. B said I could if I wanted to. Never mind wanting to, I had to. I had to see him for myself. The thing that amazed me the most about this whole situation was that Dr. B. was sitting there with an IV and a catheter and his usual big smile. I asked him how he could be smiling. Didn't he know that he could die? Wasn't he scared? This was his reply: "Scared? Why should I be scared? I have nothing to worry about. Why should I worry about dying? The Lord is with me. He is watching over me. If He wants me and it's my time to die then I'll die, and if it's not my time to die I'll live. But there is nothing I can do about it. My life is in His hands."

Several issues were critical for me. First I didn't want to lose Dr. B. He had helped me a lot and was my friend. What would I do without him? Dr. B. told me that I would be fine and that part of him was incorporated into me and I would always have that part of him. He also said that I would find another therapist if I needed one. Finding another therapist was the second critical issue. Yes, there are other doctors and yes there are other good doctors, but there are many doctors who aren't good. There are some who don't really show you that they care. Dr. B. would hug me when I left or when I was very upset. Other doctors wouldn't do that.

The bottom line is love and trust. It is difficult to trust someone with your emotional and/or physical problems. That person, the doctor, can save you or destroy you depending on his or her intelligence and competence. Speaking as someone with both emotional and physical medical problems, I have been fortunate to find doctors who are intelligent and competent and are not afraid to let me know they care about me.

I feel another critical issue is religion. I believe in God and believe that death is not the end of life but the beginning of a new and different life. Therefore, in dealing with Dr. B.'s illness, my faith has helped me and has helped him in his efforts to comfort me. That doesn't mean I won't cry or be very upset if something should happen to him, it just means that I will go on with my life and remember what he taught me and know that I will see my doctor again.

One last thought. I said to Dr. B. that sometimes I get so scared. He replied, "there's nothing to be scared of, you're not alone". He's right, God is with me.

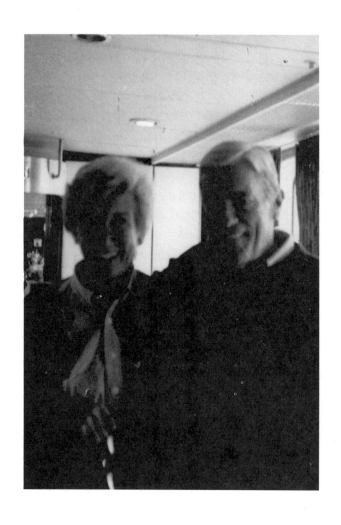

Elizabeth Warner and Silas Warner, M.D.

WAITING FOR A HEART TRANSPLANT AND BEYOND

Silas Warner, M.D

I am a retired psychiatrist, 68 years old, who moved to and has now resided in California for four years. Since moving I have been plagued by health problems stemming from chronic heart disease. My cardiac diagnosis is chronic congestive heart failure — which in itself sounds menacing and almost terminal. During the past three years I have had two open-heart operations. The first was done on June 4, 1989 and involved replacing my defective mitral valve with a new artificial (plastic) mitral valve. There was leakage around this new valve which required another open-heart surgical repair operation on October 14, 1991. The leak was successfully repaired, a pacemaker was put in my chest and I looked forward to a better, healthier life.

In January 1992, I took a few days to play golf (in a cart) in Arizona. I was having trouble breathing, felt excessively fatigued and had to return home early from my golf outing. I saw my local primary physician who told me that I now needed a heart transplant operation. Much to my alarm, I was flown in a Med-O-Vac plane on a stretcher with a nurse from the Monterey Airport to San Francisco. I was met there by an ambulance which drove me to the U.C.S.F. hospital. I went right to the intensive care cardiology unit where electronic devices were hooked up to my body. A cardiology nurse monitored this. Knowing I was in atrial fibrillation, I could follow the irregularity of my heartbeat. The electronic screen emphatically showed my heart's abnormalities.

A short while later my new cardiologist stopped by. He is an East Indian, trained in England and the United States. His competence, gentleness and patience were evident. He listened to my heart, looked at my electronic screen and told me that he thought I could be helped. He said that he would put me on the list for a heart transplant. In the meantime, he would place me on a new medical regime which he hoped would regulate my heart and substantially improve its function. I felt immediate hope and encouragement from what he said and by his unruffled, positive approach.

I was discharged with my name at the bottom of the hospital's heart transplant list. For a matching heart to become available, the usual amount of time is two to nine months. I had to carry a beeper and always be within two hours of the hospital. To make communication faster, I purchased a car phone. I have had to remain home-based in Carmel. I was placed on ten different medications, a total of 28 pills a day. I take my medication regularly five times a day and have periodic heart checkups in San Francisco.

I am limited physically and do not overexert myself, but do walk on a flat surface daily for half an hour. Much to my surprise, I was able to walk briskly for about two miles on the Carmel beach without shortness of breath. I am also allowed to play 18 holes of golf a day in a cart. I have lost 20 pounds and notice that my muscle bulk and coordination are not what they were previously. I am pleased that my weight is less and I do moderate weight-lifting exercises to improve my arm muscle tone. My appetite is sufficient, but I do not get hungry as I used to. At times I have a mildly toxic feeling which I think is from my medication. I can concentrate and read and do some writing. However, I notice that with any sustained activity such as traveling or attending a social function, I become fatigued. I still do such activities, but take naps regularly.

My cardiac checkups have been encouraging, showing both subjective and objective improvement. About two months ago I was found not to be in atrial fibrillation. I have some occasional atrial fibrillation but my heartbeat remains regular at about 80 beats per minute. A pacemaker keeps the heartbeat to a minimum of 80. My cardiologist has recently placed me on "hold" for the heart transplant list, which means that I no longer require a beeper and can travel. I am to continue having cardiac checkups, including lab work, to make certain that my prothrombin time remains stabilized. I remain on the heart transplant list, but in an inactive status. This gives me some priority should my cardiac condition worsen and I again require a heart transplant.

I first became aware of a potential heart problem in 1977 when I was suddenly hospitalized in Bryn Mawr, PA with Sub-acute Bacterial Endocarditis (SBE). All my life I have known that I had a heart murmur but was always told that it was "functional". The heart murmur did not keep me out of the Navy nor did it present any symptoms. One morning I awoke and was unable to walk because I could not keep my balance. I thought that I had had a stroke. I was rushed to the hospital's emergency room where my internist diagnosed me as having SBE. I was hospitalized and put on intravenous penicillin. My recovery was slow and was complicated by an allergy to penicillin. Having been very healthy all my life, I was not accustomed to hospital confinement. I returned home after eight weeks, having made a good recovery. Had this been before the advent of antibiotics, I would not have survived.

Until 1988 I continued my life and busy psychiatric practice as before. I then decided to retire and move to California. I had always thought that I would continue my practice indefinitely, but my financial situation was such that I could now retire. I was reluctant to leave my friends and patients in Philadelphia but with my wife's encouragement I finally made the change.

My subsequent heart problems have made me extremely thankful that I did retire in 1988. Trying to continue my psychiatric practice and deal with my cardiac problems would have been extremely difficult.

I developed a severe case of poison oak dermatitis a few months after moving to California. Little did I know that the Monterey Peninsula has been called "the poison oak capital of California". I treated myself conservatively with calamine lotion. It soon became infected and I consulted a local physician, who prescribed an oral cortisone. After listening to my heart, he ominously announced that I was in atrial fibrillation.

A cardiac consultation revealed that I had a defective mitral valve, which required an open-heart operation to replace it with an artificial plastic valve. At first it was scheduled as an elective procedure, but my condition worsened and the operation was moved to June 14, 1989. I liked my cardiac surgeon and had confidence that I would recover. Nevertheless, I was apprehensive about the six-hour surgery. I was most relieved to wake up and find that all had gone well. The operation had already been delayed for a week because my Coumadin had not been discontinued and the blood which had been set aside for the surgery could not initially be located. I experienced momentary feelings that I was "snake-bitten" and destined to have things go wrong. I received emotional support, hearing from friends who were praying for me and I said a few prayers, even though I am basically an agnostic.

I learned from this experience that I knew little about heart pathology and had to keep asking questions to learn more. My consulting cardiologist must have assumed that I was knowledgeable (being a physician) and consequently did not explain some of the basics. For example, we never discussed diet and I did not know how important it is to be on a low-salt diet. My physician did not familiarize me with the possibility of pulmonary edema and how my diuretic helped to prevent this.

While visiting in the East, I consulted another cardiologist, who thought he heard a new murmur which my California cardiologist had not heard. About a year later the murmur was louder. I was told that I needed another open-heart operation to repair the leak around my artificial mitral valve. This was discouraging.

On October 14, 1991, I had my second heart surgery with the same cardiac surgeon from California. I still had faith in him and knew that my chance for survival was better than 95%. Yet again, I was apprehensive that "bad luck" was my lot. This was in marked contrast to my usual hopeful, optimistic self. Fortunately, I went through another successful six-hour operation.

At this point I decided to change to a cardiologist at the San Jose hospital where I had the surgery. My primary cardiologist there was a little more communicative, but was in a group practice. I could never be certain that I would be able to speak to him if I phoned with a question. I had to provide other cardiologists with a detailed explanation of who I was, why I was calling, my past cardiac history and my current cardiac status. I understood that this was required, but I missed the support of a strong doctor-patient personal relationship where you did not have to explain everything every time. My cardiologist also did not make clear to me the extent of my cardiomyopathy which might require a heart transplant operation.

Knowing that alcohol consumption could kill myocardial tissue, I had stopped all drinking three years earlier. I was not an alcoholic and never missed any work due to alcohol, but I was periodically a heavy social drinker. Afraid of the consequences of additional myocardiopathy, I was strongly motivated to totally abstain from alcohol for health reasons. I did not become involved with A.A. It has been difficult never to have a drink, but I know it is critical that I do so.

How has this life-threatening experience affected me? It has totally changed my outlook and habits. It has become evident to me how precious life is and how fortunate I am to still be alive.

I have learned that I am not immortal and that I will be most fortunate to have 10 to 15 additional years of life. I spend more time now reviewing and putting in order my past life. I have reread the letters and data which my father saved from my past. I have assembled albums for my children containing pictures of them, letters, school reports, etc. This has provided a good opportunity for me to review my life and theirs. My wife is an excellent photographer and all the years of our marriage are well-documented. I do not pursue these activities in a morbid mood, but rather happily, because I now have a better perspective and can think about what it all means. I was raised as a Christian, but never became a "true believer". My only sibling, a sister, and my wife and her family are ever-stronger Christians. I wish I could have become a "true Christian believer", but my strongly scientific and rational side does not allow it. I am glad that others are so helped by Christianity and other religions. Essentially a private person, I mainly console my-self at times of crisis. I also enjoy seeing my children and grandchildren and watching how they have dealt with the everyday problems of living.

I now feel physically and emotionally ready to en-joy my remaining years. I am especially interested in reading and writing about psychobiography. I have ac-cumulated a lot of excellent material which I must now organize and write about. I am a trustee of both the York School and Planned Parenthood, both good causes. I do not want to return to psychiatric prac-tice.

My wife Libby and I have made a new start in our lives in California and enjoy the new friends, golf, and mild climate. We have a summer boathouse on Lake Cayuga in Ithaca, New York and spend two months there each summer. Our children and grandchildren live nearby. My wife and I are spending more time to-gether and are increasingly interdependent. She has been a strong and comforting companion, especially during the last few years when I have needed her. We hope to travel more, which we both enjoy. Despite my cardiac problems, I feel fortunate to be alive and feel-ing as well as I do. Without the new field of cardiac surgery, I would not have survived. Although my con-fidence was partly dependent on good physical and emotional health, I have been able to readjust to my limitations. I can no longer run, play tennis, drink alco-hol, or use much salt — but such considerations no longer seem important. My mind still functions, although my memory is noticeably poorer, but I can rationalize and say these changes accompany increasing age and are the price to be paid to survive.

Editor's Note:

On Friday, November 12, 1993, noting symptoms of worsening chronic congestive heart failure during an examination, Dr. Chatterjee increased Dr. Warner's medication dosage. Dr. Warner returned home to Carmel, spent a normal weekend, played golf on Sunday, attended the symphony Monday evening, November 15th. He suffered cardiac arrest in his sleep at 3:00 A.M. on Tuesday, November 16th. Cardio-Pulmonary Resuscitation was unsuccessful. After some fifteen to twenty minutes without oxygen, Dr. Warner was revived by 911 medics. He was subsequently flown back to University Hospital of California at San Francisco. The support systems were discontinued on Friday, November 19th. Dr. Warner died sixteen hours later on Saturday, November 20th. He never regained consciousness.

A WIFE'S PERCEPTION OF HEART DISEASE

Elizabeth Warner

I am both this essay's narrator and a physician's wife, an observer from the beginning to everything with the exception of the surgical procedures. It is because I was such a conscientious observer that I recall this period of time with anger. The anger is directed at the manner in which several doctors from the very onset mishandled my husband's medical problems. This report is not inclusive of all the shocking details of mishandling because to recall them is to be forced to relive them in excruciating detail. It was a hopelessly frustrating "Four Year Nightmare", worsened by my husband Silas L. Warner's reluctance to demand his rights or an accounting for the incredible number of mistakes, omissions and errors that were made. This was a time when I perceived minimal if any communication between doctors and was myself stonewalled by the closed-rank attitude of these same physicians.

This medical history's origin was Dr. Silas Warner's (hereinafter "Si") enlightenment as to a heart murmur during a routine insurance company physical. He was advised to take antibiotics prophylactically whenever any invasive procedure (oral surgery, deep dental cleaning, etc.) capable of introducing infection into the bloodstream through surface openings was undertaken. Considering the chances of this happening to be extremely rare, Si did not do so.

In January 1977, Si began running a low-grade fever of 99 degrees plus, which continued for several months. He appeared to be eating normally but was losing weight and had a diminished appetite. I did not think a fever should continue for such an extended period even if "Flu was going around". I urged him to get himself checked. He refused.

An excellent athlete, Si regularly played tennis in the winter and golf in the summer, yet he complained about atypically poor hand/eye coordination. He had backed out of the garage and into the fence several times.

I called my brother-in-law, a physician, stating that I thought something was wrong with my husband. My brother-in-law told me to save my breath and that if Si perceived nothing to be wrong that I was incapable of dissuading him. "That is the way doctors are." This statement would be prophetic of the next sixteen years.

In March of 1977, while letting the dogs out, Si stumbled down the hall and fell. He stated emphatically that he fell not because of a heart attack, of this he was certain. He credited the fall to poor balance resultant from an inner ear problem. While helping him back to bed, I asked if I <u>finally</u> could call a doctor. With Si's concurrence I contacted a physician, a personal friend. Our doctor advised going to the hospital by ambulance. He met us in the emergency room, examined Si briefly, suspected Subacute Bacterial Enocarditis ("SBE") but couldn't be positive without cultures. He started Si on massive IV penicillin. Cultures did show SBE. At this time Si was itching and covered with hives. I complained to the doctors and nurses; Si was allergic to penicillin. Si was switched to Keflex. He remained hospitalized for six weeks until the infection on his mitral valve was cured.

During this period of hospitalization, Si at times became quite ill - shivering, running a high fever, having difficulty keeping the thermometer in his mouth. He never mentioned these instances to the doctors or nurses and no one noticed. When these problems were ultimately addressed to the medical personnel, Si was queried as to his silence. It was the standard reply: "I didn't think it was significant."

Si made a good recovery and gradually cut back on his checkups with the cardiologist. During this time, I was not checking and took his word that his health was under control. I had always been aware that his alcohol consumption was excessive though not apparent to the public. I mentioned this but there was no positive response, only a complete denial as to any problem.

In 1986 I proposed retirement. In 1987 Si agreed to give notice for a June 1988 departure. His work seemed to be dropping off somewhat and his schedule appeared lighter. It seemed the ideal time to change the life-style of many years. We moved to California on June 1st of 1988, though Si was somewhat reluctant to move. In August our neighbors gave a welcoming party for us. Si had been running through the woods and returned home, sweating, out of breath, scratching and itching from the bushes he had run through. The bushes turned out to be poison oak and Si treated it with calamine, the poison ivy antidote. Two weeks later his lower legs and ankles were darkening and swelling badly.

I called a recommended local doctor Dr. C, who agreed to see Si immediately. Dr. C diagnosed Si's condition as poison oak, far more lethal than Eastern poison ivy. He prescribed cortisone, which was more aggressive than calamine as a poison oak treatment. Si returned in a week to be checked. Dr. C, upon listening to his heart, asked if Si was aware that he was in atrial fibrillation. Si had not noticed. Dr. C recommended consulting a cardiologist at once.

The cardiologist Dr. A examined Si, ordered medicine and remarked that a valve replacement might eventually become necessary. Dr. A performed an echogram, which I attended and personally viewed the inadequate functioning of the heart valve. Si was checked by A every six weeks through the fall of 1988 and into early 1989.

Subsequent to this period, Si seemed to fail. His color was poor and he repeatedly experienced shortness of breath. In April when Si left to do a Locum Tenens in Elmira, New York, I contacted A and related my concerns. A suggested that Si, upon his return from New York, have a stress test . This test was performed upon his arrival. I did not see this procedure but was aware that its brevity reflected Si's rapidly deteriorating condition. A suggested immediate consultation regarding a new valve with a heart surgeon. This procedure was not done in the Community Hospital.

Within a week (mid-May), we were seeing Dr. B , who said it was time to operate and for Si to start donating his own blood. Dr. B also stated that alcohol consumption was to be discontinued as the ventricle was enlarged. Surgery was scheduled for June 6, 1989.

Si arrived for heart catheterization on June 5. The cardiologist took one look and said, "You haven't stopped your Coumadin. I cannot do catheterization or you'll simply bleed out." So it was: out of the bed, out of the hospital gown, out of the hospital, cancel the surgery and back to Carmel for another week. It was hard to believe that neither the cardiologists nor the surgeon had suggested terminating the Coumadin. It was also hard to believe that my husband had not wondered about this.

The next week we returned for the rescheduled surgery. Catheterization was fine - Si had no coronary problem at all. At midnight all wristbands were removed and Si was ordered into the shower. I stated that I would not leave until the wristbands were replaced and was told that this cannot be done until the lab sends a technician for blood matching. I was also informed that the bands should not have been removed earlier by the nurse. I had questioned this removal and had been told at that time that it was "routine". At midnight with surgery scheduled for 7

AM, I asked why the blood had to be matched since Si had previously made two donations of blood expressly for the surgery. The nurse said that Si's chart did not indicate this. I then suggested that they had better check for this entry, which was eventually located.

I am not impressed with "new medicine" and can readily understand how people hospitalized for adenoids can have a leg amputated because no one knows what anyone else is doing. Everyone functions within a personal vacuum. The problem with the wristbands, exacerbated by the earlier continuation of Coumadin, made me aware of the necessity for my monitoring the entirety of Si's medical treatment.

The surgery was successful. The surgeon reported that drinking had contributed to the enlarging of Si's ventricle. The now properly working valve should, however, enable some shrinkage.

Si made a very rapid recovery but developed massive hiccups which continued for ten days. In the hospital they used old barroom techniques to cure them. None of these techniques worked. A week after surgery Si was discharged and we returned home, an hour and a half from the hospital. The hiccups were extremely debilitating. Si could not talk, eating was difficult and acupuncture was considered by Si. We knew that hiccups can occur for a period of three to four days subsequent to surgery, but ten days was very unusual.

I called a masseuse, whom I had found effective for circulation and relaxation though Si had always refused their services in the past. This time he agreed to try. The masseuse came and worked on him for an hour and a half. When Si emerged from the bedroom, the hiccups were gone. He did not mention it nor did I, lest psychologically the hiccups resume. A friend was there to witness the cessation and also said nothing. Si began the next day denying that the relaxation stopped the hiccups or improved him physically. He said that he fell asleep following the massage. When he awoke several hours later, the hiccups were gone. (Not so, they were gone immediately.) Clearly there was a conflict between taking advice from me and healing himself.

Si improved steadily and resumed normal life in July in Ithaca, New York at our summer home. It was now six weeks post-op. We had an Ithaca cardiologist Dr. Goodfriend check prothrombin levels and generally keep an eye on Si. I organized this medical monitoring as well as the transmittal of operative reports to New York. Dr. Goodfriend thought he heard a faint murmur and included this in his report to the west coast doctors, whom we saw at the end of July when we returned to California.

The California cardiologist Dr. A informed Si that he did not hear a murmur so no further tests or echograms were warranted. Si only had checkups every three months. During the fall/winter of 1989-1990, Si continued as usual, tiring a bit more easily and being out of breath more frequently, but not markedly so. We summered in Ithaca in 1990. Dr. Goodfriend continued to monitor, still felt that Si's heart was producing an increasing noise but assumed since his first observations had been relayed to the California doctors that they were cognizant of and monitoring the situation. To me Si appeared to be tiring more and more easily and was not looking very well.

We returned to Carmel at the end of the 1990 summer and Si was routinely checked by Dr. A for Coumadin. I attended all of these checkups. Si never complained though he was not sleeping well. He read for two or three hours nightly and frequently fell asleep during the day. Dr. A said everything was okay and no further tests were necessary.

By the Spring of 1991, I had become increasingly concerned. Si's skin now had a grayish cast. Dr. C took blood tests in May 1991 and later contacted us in Ithaca to advise that the blood sugar level required rechecking. Si seemed "slightly anemic, though not alarmingly so." All this had been reported to Dr. Goodfriend in anticipation of Si's July appointment.

Prior to the checkup with Dr. Goodfriend, my doctor brother-in-law advised me that Si did not look very well. My brother-in-law had questioned Si as to Dr. C's characterization of Si's condition. The reply was "chronic congestive heart failure". My brother-in-law was acquainted with the import of this condition and felt that a physical was critical. Relying on his brother's advice, Si made an appointment immediately upon our arrival in Ithaca

Dr. Goodfriend took a look and called for blood and stool tests. He also recommended a colonoscopy to determine what was causing the internal bleeding, in addition to the now very obvious leak in or around the valve resulting in hemolysis. Dr. Goodfriend also obtained permission to contact California in order to obtain Si's most recent echocardiogram. This was to be compared to the echocardiogram just taken in Ithaca. One can imagine Dr. Goodfriend's surprise (though doctors are too protective of each other and their "club" to ever let anyone know their surprise) when advised that the last echocardiogram dated back two and a half years!

Dr. Goodfriend wrote a four-page report inclusive of his findings and recommendations which he forwarded to Drs. C and A. He also said in a separate letter to C that, "Dr. and Mrs. Warner are not completely satisfied with the cardiac treatment and might possibly be seeking new doctors." He added that he had suggested a larger center such as Stanford or San Francisco.

We saw Dr. A the day after our return from the East. He came into the office, as usual late, and remarked, "Don't I have a letter somewhere from someone about you?" We said that he did. Dr. A then sat down, opened a file and read silently for a considerable time what was obviously Dr. Goodfriend's very detailed thorough report. It was quite obvious to me, as is was to Si, that this was Dr. A's first exposure to the medical report. Dr. A did not comment on the content of the report. He just said, "Let's have a listen" and "I think it's time to get up to see Dr. B , sounds very noisy, etc., etc., I'll call him at once." Dr. A never referred to Dr. Goodfriend's report. He never made the customary comment, i.e. "Yes, I agree" or "I hear something" and "we do need to check things" or "something has changed". He never made any statement that indicated his response to another doctor's recommendations.

52

The following week we had a trans-esophageal echocardiogram ("TEE") with Dr. D. (Dr. D is one of eight cardiologists on a team, all of whom we were going to get to know, though not one of them would know Si very well.) Dr. Goodfriend had specifically recommended a TEE because the ordinary echo tends to have a shadow cast by the artificial valve. Dr. D did the TEE. He later confirmed that a leak existed. Stitches were loose but it was uncertain whether the tissue simply gave way or the stitches had been wrenched out. It didn't matter. The stitches needed to be repaired and the sooner the better.

Dr. D immediately sent a report to Dr. B (surgeon) and we saw B soon after. It intrigues me how rapidly doctors respond when they think they may be held accountable. All kinds of doors are almost miraculously opened. It can be done, but at what cost in every way!

An appointment was made for a gastroenterologist, who scheduled a colonoscopy for the next week, to ascertain the cause of bleeding distinct from bleeding resultant from crushing in the valve. B said he would operate upon clearance from the gastroenterologist. There was no discussion about Si and autologous blood. I guess there wasn't time.

During the colonoscopy, they discovered a sizeable tumor, six centimeters, which they were able to get with the scope. The danger of perforating the colon was discussed since the tumor was so close to the wall. The risk of major abdominal surgery preceding major heart surgery was judged to be greater than that of perforation. They were successful. The cardiac surgeon was elated and was willing to proceed. This series of events transpired between mid-September and early October of 1991.

On October 15, 1991, Dr. B operated, shored up stitches and stated, "These will NEVER come loose." I refrained from asking why they had previously become loosened. Si recovered rapidly and without attendant hiccups. We decided to use the cardio-team rather than Dr. A for regular checkups, general monitoring medication and the installation of a pacemaker.

At this time, I called Dr. A.'s office and requested that copies of Si's medical records be sent to our home. The office agreed to this. Three weeks later the records had not arrived. I went to the office and obtained them. In the car I examined the documents that had been given me and discovered that Dr. Goodfriend's report was missing. Si, though shocked at this seemingly deliberate omission, did not press the issue.

Si returned for a checkup a month later with Dr. B. Dr. B was amazed at Si's recovery which contrasted emphatically with "everything rattling around inside, in such a bad state of disrepair that it had to have been going on for some time and didn't just happen in the last few weeks." I was apprehensive, because I was intimidated by doctors, about questioning why Si's medical problems had not previously been so glaringly apparent. The questions were never asked and so this matter was unresolved.

Si was fine until Thanksgiving 1991, approximately six weeks after surgery, when he noticed a fluid buildup in his legs. He attributed this condition to the long interval spent working at his desk. I asked if he should call a doctor but he declined. By the next day there was a greater accumulation of fluid and Si was slightly short of breath. He spoke with one of the physicians and his dosage of Lasix was increased. The swelling in his ankles abated.

We traveled to New York City for medical meetings in early December. Si was very enervated and napped throughout the day. We departed from New York and proceeded to California to see Dr. E, a member of the "Team". Dr. E viewed the situation as fine. By Thursday, December 12 at around midnight, Si was standing, couldn't breathe, forbade my calling a doctor and ultimately slept in a sitting position. In the morning, with Si's concurrence, I contacted the doctors who recommended increasing the Lasix.

I then contacted Dr. C, who had Dr. F on-call. Dr. F, who had a cursory report of Si's condition, asked for a chest X-ray which showed a tiny speck of fluid in the bottom corner of the lung. F's solution was more Lasix. F became annoyed when I suggested that his solution did not address the problem. Si was of no assistance - stating, "Oh, leave it alone. You don't know what you're talking about." What I do know is that gasping for breath is indicative of an emergency.

Si saw Dr. B two days later at a social affair. B clapped Si on the shoulder and commented as to how well he looked. I listened as B, arm over Si's shoulder, pontificated to the surrounding guests saying, "This is my prize patient, snaps back like a rubber band, etc., etc." Everyone oohed and ahhed but I sensed that Si was very ill. Si did not, however, terminate B's congratulations nor self-aggrandizement by stating, "Actually, just last week I had a very severe setback of some sort." No way.

Si's health was noticeably deteriorating. The fluid buildups were becoming frequent occurrences. When Si experienced another attack, I called another team man and he says, "More Lasix." I offered to drive Si but the doctor viewed this as too dangerous. The doctor suggested going to a nearby emergency room, where I realized the staff would be ignorant as to Si's medical history. Finally I contacted another team doctor Dr. E, who was annoyed, not on duty and didn't speak pleasantly. I admittedly can be annoying, a trait doubtlessly intensified by the continuing severity of my husband's condition. I was eventually told to call back at 9 AM, when the office opened and make an appointment . For once Si intervened and said, "Let's simply go up there and be there when the office opens and maybe that will have some effect."

Si saw the doctor at 11 AM. The doctor said that all seemed to be going well due to the increased Lasix and abstinence from salt. A lengthy lecture on salt and its multiple adverse effects followed, though Si has never overused salt. This lecture was the first time that salt had been mentioned to Si. It appeared that we were viewed as entirely culpable for the fluid buildup. After the speech, I commented that Si's ankle had swollen slightly. Dr. E's comment was, "Oh, that's unrelated!" I wanted to ask, "Unrelated to what?", but I didn't ask. I was once again intimidated and Si would be annoyed at "petty" or "sarcastic" questions.

When we departed for Ithaca for the Christmas holidays, things seemed to be under control though Si's health seemed to have regressed (in my eyes and opinion) since Thanksgiving. Christmas necessitated a minimum of effort and plenty of rest and escape from holiday family confusion for Si. We left Ithaca on December 29. On January 3, 1992 there was a scheduled appointment with Dr. E, who characterized the situation as fine. Another echo would not, therefore, be required for several months. Si mentioned his decreasing appetite but E assured him that time would solve that.

We left for Arizona for five-day golf trip. Si was feeling so ill that he played only nine holes and had great difficulty retaining food. The first night Si had a violent attack, gasping for breath and hanging over the sink. I called Dr. E's office and was advised that he was not on-call. I repeated that this was an emergency; I had to deal exclusively with Dr. E and that it was critical that he contact me as soon as possible. Dr. E returned the call an hour later and suggested increasing the Lasix and making an appointment upon our return. I do not understand what others define as an "emergency" but Si was in acute distress. It was not until the next day that this acute stage was over.

We arrived at our Carmel home on Monday, January 13 and called Dr. C to schedule a Tuesday appointment. After his examination, Dr. C said that Si should be hospitalized to have his medication successfully regulated. Dr. C said, "Knowing how you feel about the cardiologist (A) here, I will get another cardiologist to walk you through the procedure." Si still considered Dr. C to be preferable and returned home with medicine to self-administer. I strongly felt that Si should be hospitalized. Reluctantly he contacted Dr. C and entered the hospital that day, Tuesday the 14th. On Wednesday January 15, medication IV was started to regulate his heart. Si was to be monitored by Dr. G, an older cardiologist and a member of A's group.

As of Wednesday afternoon when I had returned home, I had not been apprised of Si's condition by either Dr. C or Dr. G. Si telephoned stating, "Dr. C and Dr. G have just told me my only hope is a heart transplant." I was momentarily stunned by this news.

I rushed back to the hospital, where I was introduced to Dr. G, an affable older man in his seventies. He informed us of the existence of heart transplant centers. Dr. B knew a surgeon. Si might be too old for one of these transplant centers though yet another center "takes 'em one year older than he is." We all laughed politely at this joke among the cardiac surgeons. Dr. G said it would be advisable to make the decision expeditiously so that he could start the wheels turning before the weekend. I thought, "wow they're in one big hurry to get the responsibility of Si off their backs!"

We asked Dr. G for information on several subjects that would influence our decision: There was a rumor that Dr. Chatterjee of UCSF was going on sabbatical. We had contact with one hospital through Dr. B, what about that? What is the age situation at another hospital? Dr. G said these concerns would be discussed first thing on Thursday morning at 8 AM. Si asked me to be very prompt, no walking to the hospital. I arrived precisely at 8 AM and we commenced waiting. We asked for Dr. G (Si did so grudgingly, unwilling to be a "bother" to a busy doctor); we were told G was in the hospital overseeing stress tests. Another hour went by and we were informed that he had left the hospital. At eleven, after a three hour wait, my patience, unlike Si's, was nonexistent and I went home.

Si telephoned and announced that he was being taken by ambulance to UCSF and Dr. Chatterjee. He stated that it was all arranged and he required a few things. I returned to the hospital and was informed that a helicopter had been dispatched since it was illegal to use an ambulance for that distance. I returned home again, got more things and went to the airport. I arrived at the airport and saw a Med-Evac twin engine plane. Si, all IV's attached, was aboard with two nurses. According to FAA regulations, I could not accompany Si. I was only allowed on the plane for a minute to speak with him. My option was to drive 120 miles to San Francisco and meet him there.

I drove alone to the hospital and went to the Coronary Intensive Care Unit where Si had been installed and attached to dozens of monitors. Two nurses were constantly in attendance, adjusting the monitors and providing an astonishing amount of care and knowledge. Si was looking remarkably relaxed and already appeared to be improving. He must have felt that something was very wrong. This environment was going to improve his state! Within three days Si had recuperated dramatically. He remained in the hospital for an additional week and continued to improve steadily under the remarkable and thorough care of Dr. Chatterjee. Dr. Chatterjee's expertise was soon apparent through the many accolades that my research revealed. Unfortunately several months before Si had elected not to consult this doctor.

The staff at San Francisco were astounded that Si had never been given nitroglycerin during obviously emergency situations, where the valve had been leaking, acute attacks had taken place and there was an inability to breathe. We left the hospital with dozens of medications plus nitroglycerin for an emergency. Si would become an outpatient, waiting with beepers and car phones for the announcement of an available heart.

On January 29 we and the assortment of alert equipment returned home. Si reacted poorly to halcyon. In the middle of the night he fell down a flight of stairs and broke his collarbone. Dr. James, an orthopedist, examined him and said the crack was self-healing. A week later Si was admitted to the hospital complaining of severe pain under the lower rib cage. He didn't think it was appendicitis since his had been removed. Dr. C saw him and said that it was probably a gall bladder attack, which could be X-rayed the next day. In the meantime, considering the valve, Si was put on prophylactic antibiotics. The gastroenterologist indicated the possibility of gall bladder surgery.

I alerted Dr. Chatterjee as to the latest developments and he asked me to have the local doctors make sure that Si had not thrown a clot somewhere in the intestines. Chatterjee had to go through me, which seemed like an insane way to conduct medicine.

The next day Si waited for an extended period of time for the X-ray which eventually occurred but no results were given. Si was feeling better and the pain had started to diminish. In the late afternoon the gastroenterologist came in and announced that the abdomen was absolutely clear. They had taken a chest X-ray which revealed a tiny spot of fluid in the lungs, which could produce pain under the rib. The antibiotics had remedied this situation. Released from the hospital, Si returned to his previous position that I was an alarmist, seeing and hearing inaccurately, making much ado about nothing. There was no point in pursuing this subject.

Si continued to improve and Dr. Chatterjee passed over three heart donors. He saw Si monthly, continued to regulate his medication levels and finally informed us that Si had miraculously recovered. He gave Si the best possible report, short of removing Si's name from the transplant list. The heart transplant was put on indefinite hold.

We are finally liberated from the two-hour tether to UCSF. We flew eastward where Si checked in with the Ithaca cardiologist Dr. Goodfriend, who was the first to blow and continued to blow a series of whistles that demanded attention. It was the response to this demand for attention that enabled Si to happily play golf on a regular basis and more importantly to enjoy good health.

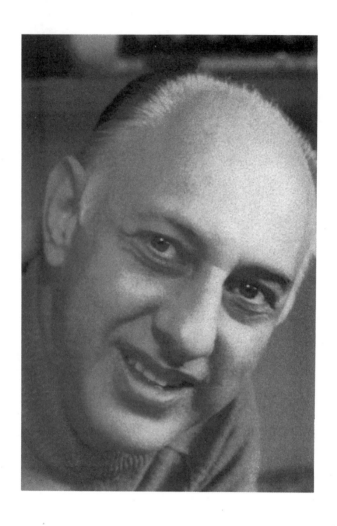

Lester A. Gelb, M.D.

A PSYCHIATRIST WITH CARDIAC PROBLEMS

Lester A. Gelb, M.D.

Transference & Countertransference Considerations

In 1952 while serving as a psychiatrist in a large rehabilitation center, I was called to see a man Hans Schoenberner. Schoenberner was the editor of a famous European satire and commentary magazine *Simplissimus*. The medical staff considered him to be mentally disordered. He had remained jovial after he had survived a criminal assault which left him a quadriplegic. "Ah, a manic," I thought. He wasn't. He smiled and seemed composed. I told him why I was seeing him. He said, "Look, if I were a football player I'd really be in trouble because I'd have to find another career. But I am one of those despised intellectuals. I use my head and I still have my head."

Our encounter turned out to be one of the most memorable in my career. I asked him what I could do for him. He answered, "I can move my right hand. Get the orthopods to rig up a support for my right arm so it can be suspended over a typewriter. I will do the rest." I did what he requested. His soon to be published book was entitled <u>You Still Have Your Head</u>. Its subject was not his physical condition though he certainly used his head. The book conveyed his perceptions of world conditions. Schoenberner subsequently wrote and published several more books and periodically reviewed books for *The New York Times*. Many years later the message that he conveyed so forcefully through his personality and his works would sustain me through difficult times.

In 1970 I had a heart attack. I had bypass surgery in 1975 and in 1986. These episodes interrupted an ongoing psychiatric and psychoanalytic practice. My patients and I had to deal not only with an unexpected hiatus in therapy but with the implications of being in therapy with an analyst who had a life-threatening condition. These matters had to be dealt with. It was, and is, critical that both my patients and myself be clear about the feelings, behavior and ideas referable to them and the effect on the therapeutic process. The patient depends on the therapeutic process to overcome suffering. A threat to that process will invariably produce significant anxiety. This is compounded by the fear of permanent loss.

My circumstances have inspired several of my colleagues to raise vexing questions about my therapeutic relationship with my patients: The medical and surgical events you have experienced and the cardiac condition you live with must produce powerful transference reactions from your patients. How do you deal with these? Haven't you experienced a significant countertransference which it is difficult for you to resolve?

Why are these questions so vexing? First, I have always been uneasy about the use of the terms transference and countertransference. They have become increasingly ambiguous. Second, the questions imply that because I have a cardiac condition, patients will react to me with stronger feelings and that my own reactions will be difficult to handle.

Reviewing the various concepts of transference and countertransference promulgated in literature, it quickly becomes apparent that there is disagreement among analysts and schools of analysis as to the exact nature of these terms. We are all familiar with the theory, originating with Freud, that transference refers to feelings for the analyst that are derived from forgotten childhood feelings toward the parents in the Oedipal period. The origin of these feelings are unconscious and there is a compulsion to repeat them. These feelings can be made conscious through interpretation by an analyst, who is neutral and anonymous. The analyst functions as a mirror allowing the patient to project his or her own subjective processes onto the analyst. By contrast Racker (1968) in his insightful *Transference and Countertransference*, noting that Freud frequently advised against relating facts of the analyst's life to patients, wrote: "Be a mirror thus meant 'speak to the patient only of himself.' It did not mean, 'stop being of flesh and blood and transform yourself into glass covered with silver nitrate.' (p. 31)

Lasky's "Catastrophic Illness in the Analyst and the Analyst's Emotional Reaction to It" addresses the author's own experience with catastrophic illness. He has a classical Freudian analytic practice in which the therapist's anonymity is a requisite to protect the transference. Lasky courageously struggled to carry out the profoundly difficult task of maintaining such a stance after his sudden need for surgery.

Questions invariably arise. Does not the analyst speak of himself by his very manner of being? Can a mirror-like stance be maintained if the analyst has an observable illness? My experience with my first analyst is pertinent here. He was someone analyzed by Freud, someone who greeted me prior to each session in a warm, smiling, even affectionate manner. He sat behind the analytic couch, supposedly non-intrusive, yet his every movement, the depth and rhythm of his breathing, his quiet chuckles or suppressed laughter all communicated his feelings and his reactions to what I was saying or doing. I sensed his subjective state as separate from our interaction.

One day his posture when entering his office was less than erect. Behind my couch I could sense that he was bent forward and that his breathing was less regular than customary. I stopped speaking and said, "Perhaps we shouldn't go on now. Are you in pain?" He answered, "I should have said something. OK, we'll continue next time." That was not to be the case as he had to recover from an appendectomy. My wife and I did not consider ourselves "intrusive" when we sent him roses during his recuperation nor was he "intrusive" when he thanked me and said that the gift was appreciated. (Years later, in 1970, when I had a heart attack, he did the same when he visited me in the hospital.)

It has long seemed apparent to me that neutrality is an impossibility. Yet many analysts attempt it. During my analytic training, patients and analysts were uncomfortable, even phobic, about the possibility of accidentally meeting in a social or casual situation. Many analysts remember those times! The rule of distancing and anonymity even seemed to be accepted by the lay culture. One day when I was joyfully wheeling my baby daughter down the street, I was accosted by the local pharmacist. Wise in the ways of Freud, he said disparagingly, "An analyst should not be seen pushing a baby carriage!"

Since Freud's original depiction of transference and countertransference, many leaders in the psychoanalytic field have offered alternatives to these concepts, especially the rule of neutrality. Stolorow et al (1987) would expunge the rules of abstinence and neutrality and emphasized a "sustained empathic inquiry." (p. 43) They perceived transference as "...an expression of the continuing influence of organizing principles and imagery that crystallized out of the patient's early formative experiences." (p. 36)

Kaufman (1956) quoting Freud, "The peculiarity of the transference lies in its excess in both character and degree over what is rational and justifiable." Kaufman redefines transference as, "The distorted and the irrational as expressed toward the analyst." He further rejects Freud's construct that transference refers to "...the replacement of a former person by the physician." (p.209) Kaufman believes that transference behavior is in the here and now and that countertransference serves as a way to maintain isolation and detachment of the patient from the therapist and the therapeutic goal of change. (p. 210)

In *The Psychiatric Interview* Sullivan never used the specialized concept of transference but instead employed the term "parataxic distortion" to refer to the persistent presumption that a person in the present will act like a significant other person from the past. (p. 231)

Bonime (1989) views the concept of transference as neither convincing nor useful. He feels that the concept "clouds rather than dynamically illuminating important aspects of personality and their functioning in analysis." and that "...employing the constructs of transference and countertransference unnecessarily convolutes and hinders exploration of the patient and the reciprocal personal impacts during the clinical process." (p.376)

Case studies in the classical Freudian model seem limited in scope because of the focus on transference. For example, Merton Gill, author of *Analysis of Transference* emphasizes that analysis of transference must have primacy and priority. (p. 57) He has developed what he believes to be a new, more consistent and systematic elaboration of transference in therapy and with Irwin Hoffman illustrates this ideology with nine audio-recorded sessions. While reading these transcripts, I was troubled by the therapists' seemingly aggressive and intrusive pursuit of the patient. Almost every feeling and reaction of the patient vis-a-vis other people was ascribed to patient-therapist trans-ference. A potential consequence of this single-minded approach is to ignore the full scope and nature of the pa-tients' relationship with other important people in their lives. Adhering to this model, a therapist's visible illness could provoke additional transference resulting in further diminution of therapeutic freedom.

Does a chronic illness, such as cardiac disease, reduce the therapist's ability to provide optimal treatment? This question is addressed to some extent by Witenberg (1979). He considers that any distraction from total focus on the needs of the patient ascribable to the therapist's needs may be labeled countertransference. (pp. 47-48) He notes that vicissitudes of life, inclusive of health problems, can be dealt with but may sometimes overload the analytic process. (p. 48)

A colleague retired from practice after a heart attack. Although otherwise symptom free, he developed intoler-able tension and occasional arrhythmia when conducting sessions. By contrast, although depressed and frustrated by my post-hospitalization physical limitations, I was eager to resume my practice and felt relaxed with patients. I have experienced, since my initial heart attack, various physical discomforts attributable to other conditions. At times I have been sorry I scheduled a patient even wishing for a cancellation. Nevertheless, I am almost never sorry once a session begins, becoming fully absorbed and actually more comfortable after seeing a patient.

Witenberg (1979) also describes this feeling: "For many it is a relief to be able to see patients at times like these, to recognize that although one is helpless about some events in one's life it does not interfere with the ability to attend properly to one's patients. It is helpful and to some extent healing to be able to know that one can work, that one's professional identity is intact," (p. 48) I believe it is also healing for the patients.

Lasky (1990) notes that literature pertaining to catastrophic illness in a therapist is sparse. He found only 17 germane references. He wonders why this is so since Freud himself, the most prominent of analysts, suffered a catastrophic illness.

How did Freud deal with his own catastrophic illness? Much can be ascertained from Peter Gay's work Freud - A Life of Our Time. Freud diagnosed his own condition. At first he kept the diagnosis secret from his doctors, fearing that he would have to give up his addiction to smoking. Only after his cancer had progressed to the point where surgery was required (in 1923, the first of more than 30 operations) did he confide in a few intimates. (pp. 418-419) By 1927 he had periods of bitterness and depression and a sense of "decrepitude" which disillusioned him. (p. 525) He also had periods of angina. His hearing was affected by surgery, so he had to move his couch to another wall to present his better ear. (p. 427) Freud persisted, however, in writing his literary masterpieces and in seeing new patients until the year before his death. (p. 427)

I spoke with a colleague, now 83, who was analyzed by Freud in 1930. I asked him how he had reacted to Freud's illness, if the illness interfered with the analysis and what, if anything, Freud communicated about his condition. My colleague recalled that Freud's speech was quite intelligible and that he did not appear disabled. Freud did occasionally appear uncomfortable with his mouth prosthesis and frequently adjusted it. Freud said little about his condition. "He was very much task oriented." My informant recalled that he had not been worried about Freud's health nor did he believe others were because "they came to get help for their own troubles." He did recall, however, having a dream in which Freud was seriously ill. In analyzing the dream Freud made a passing allusion to his own illness but primarily focused on other significant aspects of the dream.

There was a brief item after I had an accident when I came into the office with a crutch. Most patients asked what had happened and I answered them. We then proceeded with the collaborative work of the therapy. A few patients initially said nothing. Their later questions revealed that they wanted to be reassured that my crutch did not impact on my ability to assist them.

One of my most difficult patients came to me after her previous psychiatrist had terminated his practice due to a heart attack. She is a 50 year old woman, who has always lived a severely constricted life in a hostile dependent relationship with her parents. She is agoraphobic, somewhat improved by therapy, but remains with multiple phobias, adamantly self-protected by ingenious avoidances. She still uses her former therapist as a foil. For example, "You expect too much from me, you don't understand me like my other doctor did." When cardiac surgery required my prolonged absence, she was the only patient to whom I did not tell the nature of my illness. In fact she requested that I not tell her, saying, "Whatever it is, don't tell me, just let me know about when you'll be back and give me the name of someone to fill in for you." She never called the person I had arranged for her to see. My other patients were provided with a simple explanation as to my absence, but in this instance I did allow a patient to be shielded from the implication of my condition. I was influenced by her expressed and unexpressed wishes and from her profound emotional retardation. That does not mean that I did not challenge her in other areas. I have concentrated on helping her make excursions from her home, graduate from a community college, shop alone and volunteer as a companion at a center for physically disabled adults.

Another difficult though always intriguing patient was in marked contrast to the aforementioned patient. This 40 year old successful executive had learned techniques of manipulation from his father and uncles. He was adept at insistent good natured cajoling. In therapy he had been able to relinquish a great deal of what we termed his "king complex." This patient made the ultimate confrontation with my heart surgery.

The night before my surgery he located, probably under pressure of anxiety, my hospital and my room.   When he observed that I was intact, he first seemed relieved and then acutely embarrassed. He stiffened and grandiloquently announced, "I came here not to intrude, but merely to let you know that if there is anything in the world you might need, you only have to call and ask." He left immediately when I responded, "Hello, Paul, I'll be OK. See you later."

Should I have been outraged at this intrusion? At that time I didn't want to think of psychodynamics. In retrospect I was glad to see him because it is lonely on a cardiac unit. His appearance underscored my connection with others. When I returned to therapy he apologized profusely. The subsequent examination of the incident illustrated a reversal of roles and his assumption of power. This was an inherent part of his growth and change.

A third patient, a robust man of 65 who had single-handedly been constructing on weekends a summer house, reported chest pains to me prior to advising his family physician. The patient was insistent that I refer him to a competent cardiologist. When I did, he chose another cardiologist. He explained later that upon evaluating my recovery he had second thoughts. My recovery was not synonymous with the absolute cure that he was seeking. This patient ultimately responded very well to cardiac medication and was soon symptom free, although subject to occasional arrhythmia. I assisted him in realizing that he could not continue a pattern of such heavy labor.

My reactions to this patient are pertinent He, unlike me, was symptom free, robust and able to tolerate and use advantageously certain medications. I envied him his healthy appearance. Many patients have said to me upon their arrival, "Hello, you're looking very good today," which accentuates my infirm appearance. Certainly I desire to be invulnerable or at least to slough off difficulties. This does not preclude me from experiencing pleasure at my patient's resilience and concern for the self-destructive pathology for which I treat him.

I don't believe envy is pathological unless it creates dysfunctional tension or interferes with a relationship. Don't we all envy the dancer's ability to leap or the jazz musician's ability to improvise? Yet on a reciprocal level, I know that some of my patients are glad that my illness is exclusively mine and not theirs. One patient, a narcissistic, hypercritical, comfort-seeking 68 year old woman told me she had developed a blood disorder. She stated, "I used to be jealous of you because you had such a facility with words and superior to you because I was healthy. Now I can't feel superior to you anymore."

Some patients were glad to hear that I had a cardiac history. These people were not motivated by malice. They viewed my medical history as a basis for greater empathy with their varied problems. An extremely intelligent, well-informed 57 year old woman sought help for a post-traumatic stress disorder. She had sustained a broken shoulder as a result of an accident at her place of business. I believe her neurosis was provoked because her security and well-being were dependent on her employer's high opinion of and reliance on her. By contrast in other relationships, with her husband, children and parents, she had always been taken for granted. Her anxiety and depression snowballed when her employers fired her because she could no longer type. Working with her I strove to help her develop a less dependent sense of self. I was careful to analyze all tendencies on her part to cast me in an idealized role. I never withheld my concern and understanding for her plight, including her anger at the social inequities involved in her job loss.

This patient eventually shared a carefully guarded secret. She had years earlier undergone cardiac surgery. Her reluctance to tell me was due to her fear that if I "knew all," I would be incapable of accepting and helping her. I would perceive her as "too far gone - too much to handle." I wondered if she would be able to accept my condition! When I shared my cardiac history with her she was delighted, saying that I would be able to understand her better and would serve as a model through my ability to function. It came to pass that she had another opportunity to share a malady with me. I had an accident and broke my shoulder. Would she be "delighted" when I next saw her. After the requisite hospitalization, I was released. My patient seemed genuinely concerned but also amazed that I could write and function so well with a broken arm. This encouraged her to do more work around the house, to baby-sit her new grandchild and to obtain computer programming training.

I don't suggest that a disability will make one a more effective therapist. I do believe that both patients and therapists are subject to the positive and negative vicissitudes of life. The shared realization of this fact enables rather than disables the therapeutic process.

CODA

I hope I have answered some of the questions concerning how patients and therapists are affected by a history of catastrophic illness or by the presence of catastrophic illness or disability sustained by the therapist. These reactions may be fueled by past or present experiences unrelated to the therapeutic relationship. Each patient is influenced by a multitude of factors: family history, cultural bias, societal values and his previous or current exposure to his own illness or that of others. It would not be valid or beneficial to label these reactions with the technical terms, transference or countertransference, however they may be defined.

It has been twenty years since my heart attack. Any perception patients may have as to my condition does not interfere with my therapeutic efficacy or their involvement in our collaboration. Some may have reactions, overt, subtle or hidden; these reactions are dealt with. Illness, disability and aging are the realities of the continuum of the lives of all of us. Our lives are worthy of the struggle often required to sustain the quality of life.

Editor's Note:

Dr. Gelb passed away on May 7, 1994 with a diagnosis of myocardial infarction (heart attack) An autopsy report, however, revealed that he died from a different ailment. His death was accompanied by extreme difficulty in breathing. The autopsy indicated Hamman-Rich syndrome, idiopathic interstitial fibrosis of the lungs. This syndrome is also called fibrosing alveolitis. Another name for this condition is interstitial pneumonia of Liebow, a progressive inflammatory condition starting with diffuse alveolar damage and resulting in fibrosis and honeycombing over a variable time period; also a common feature of collagen-vascular diseases.

BIBLIOGRAPHY

Bonime, W. (1989), *Collaborative Psychoanalysis*, Fairleigh Dickinson University Press, Rutherford, NJ

Gay, P. (1988), *Freud - A Life of Our Time*, W.W. Norton & Company, New York, NY

Gill, M. (1982), *Analysis of Transference*, Vol. I & II (with Hoffman, I.Z.), International Universities Press, Inc., New York, NY

Kaufman, S.S. (1956), "Countertransference", *Psychotherapy: Journal of the Robbins Institute*, 1:3, pp. 209-220

Lasky, R. (1990), "Catastrophic Illness in the Analyst and the Analyst's Emotional Reaction to It", *International Journal of Psycho-Analysis*, 71:

Racker, H. (1968), *Transference and Countertransference*, International University Press, Inc., New York, NY

Stolorow, R.D., Grandchaft, B., Atwood, G.E. (1987), *Psychoanalytic Treatment, an Intersubjective Approach*, The Analytic Press, Hillsdale, NJ

Sullivan, H.S. (1954), *The Psychiatric Interview*, W.W. Norton & Company, Inc., New York, NY

Witenberg, E.G. (1979), "The Inner Experience of the Psychoanalyst", In: Epstein, L. and Feiner, A.H., Eds., *Countertransference*, Jason Aronson, Inc., New York, NY

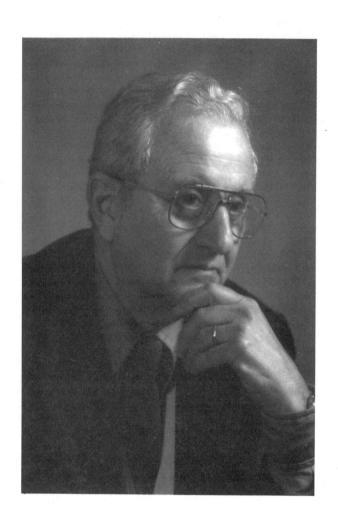

Irvin A. Kraft, M.D.

DOUBLE-BLIND GUINEA PIG

Irvin A. Kraft, M.D.

Good medical research fascinates and tugs on some of us to participate, even as subjects. I volunteered for the Physicians Health Study at its very beginning, sometime in the late seventies. I truly believed and felt this constituted a noble project in which I could identify with being a physician and a contributor to medical science. I faithfully followed their directions using two sets of pills, one for betacarotene and the other for aspirin. My peers and age-mates in pediatrics and internal medicine commented that they took aspirin daily and asked me what my regimen was. "No, I cannot break the protocol, my covenant with the project."

In 1986 I awakened in the middle of the night with severe dyspepsia. I tried to no avail my usual, workable routine of Tums and a carbonated drink. I speculated as to the possibility of an infarction but dismissed this idea.

I was in full, complete denial. I went to my so-called health club, realized that I was much more tired than usual yet proceeded to my office for a thirteen hour workday. A feeling of atypical fatigue persisted. That night in a conversation with my internist and close friend, I mentioned my concern about my cardiac condition; I was scheduled to go on a scuba diving trip in the near future. He suggested that I see him in his office the next morning. That morning I parked my car at the School of Public Health and briskly walked a half-mile across campus to my doctor's office.

An EKG put me into a wheelchair. Within an hour I underwent an arteriorgram and enzyme studies. These tests revealed in no uncertain terms that I had efficiently blocked a small branch of the left coronary artery. A day later from the acute coronary care unit I called the Physicians Health Study in Boston. In response to my query I was told: "Yes, you were on a placebo."

With my genetics - both parents and an older sister succumbed to arteriosclerotic heart disease, how could I have risked so much for those vaunted feelings of oneness with the other physician-subjects and my so-called contributions to medical science? Was the donation of my myocardiogram worth that much? Denial enveloped me and recriminations soared. My sense of invincibility had been enhanced by regular exercise, jogging, tennis, cholesterol never excessive, no diabetes, never smoking, minimal alcohol consumption and 40-year weight maintenance. My invincibility crumbled to tiny bits of deep disappointment. Silent ischemia became my ever present, shrouded companion.

My heart and I presented ourselves to the standard procedures of arteriograms (6 or 7), angioplasties (3), rehabilitation, an assortment of calcium blockers and on-and-on. I felt more was needed and I tracked down the local PET center. This cardiac Lorelei beckoned and I managed to enlist my heart in their protocol. At this time my first angioplasty had re-stenosed within six months and I dwelled in the shadow of the second, which lasted 2 1/2 years. A third one did not illicit much optimistic fervor. During this period my cardiologist and internist had not breathed a word about PET scans as a means of better understanding my status. I had become in a very standardized, very accepted fashion, a "guinea pig".

What did this not uncommon cardiac sequence mean in the light of a less common placebo role for humanity? I felt that I had betrayed myself and my own self-interests. By not taking aspirin I had begun a long winding trail and sequence to experiences, tests, expenditures and ultimately bypass surgery with rather severe secondary consequences, such as intense, chronic idiopathic bilateral edema and significant weight gain. Now, did I feel noble, dedicated and generous?

How do others in serious, double-blind studies feel? After all I had performed such clinical research for over ten years with psychopharmacologic agents for children without any real contemplation of what this meant to my child patients and their families. I knew then that with the very limited resources available in my community that at least these families got some workup and attention. There were often surprisingly positive results. How could I now rationalize tests dependent on placebos? Was the foregoing conclusion enough to go on without further questioning? Researchers claim that the gold standard for clinical research is the double-blind procedure. Is this fair to the patient?

Obviously I had an insignificant response to the placebo, since my coronary arteries kept right on occluding. In behavioral studies the placebo responses can be up to 40% positive. How do I differentiate in my case? Did I have some sort of belief that the study was only going to reinforce and augment my imperviousness? Perhaps I suspected that it would keep my fate at bay - my father had a silent coronary at 64 and I was 64 1/2! In my guinea pig status I competed to survive my father, who ultimately died of a massive infarction at age 77.

A placebo-revelation carries with it a melange of feelings. Some feelings exist on the surface while others lurk and influence the total response. In summary, BEWARE OF DOUBLE-BLIND participation until you search yourself several times. To be or not to be the guinea pig - that becomes the question.

Traditionally physicians make poor patients for a variety of reasons. Knowledge of what could go wrong tempers any great enthusiasm to make one's doctor into the omnipotent transferential positive father figure, as the typical patient is inclined to do. "What if?" may dominate the physician's thinking, leading to an internal struggle of: should I believe what he says? Should I get a second opinion? Or, maybe it will recede, just go away, if I ignore it longer?

Adaption to a role assignment requires time. A physician undergoes 5 to 8 or more years having his thinking and deportment molded and shaped by medical school and specialty training. My favorite illustration of this point occurred when several of us third year medical students were lounging at the medical clinic entrance awaiting patients. Dr. Elaine Rossi frowning advanced towards us and forcibly, bluntly said, "A doctor doesn't stand with his hands in his pockets!"

Part of the medical molding process includes obtaining emotional distance from the patient and his illness. How many tales have been narrated by doctors of their experiences as a patient and the mixture of feelings and emotions aroused by that episode. This humbling experience can lead to a departure from emotional distance to a greater empathic communication with his own patients. Then how does he look for this from his own doctor and still communicate his fears, doubts and his awareness of possible wayward events?

Picture a doctor's situation when confronted with being part of a double-blind study. How can he utilize his physician role model and reconcile it with the giving up of his power to the research design? The essence of his performance, his self-image lays in the doctor-patient relationship which is now reversed (when is it to be restated as the patient-doctor relationship?).

In psychiatry we insist that the person seeking our help be termed a patient, not a client and certainly not a consumer. Doctors do not achieve equanimity as providers. Thus, power over one's self-image becomes involved on several levels inclusive of how one assumes and lives out the role of "patient". Patient status places the doctor in the dependent position, meaning non-powerful. He then visualizes himself in the system in which he had occupied an elitist role and now is reduced to being the subject of procedures, of strange personnel and of rules and regulations that effectively demoralize and diminish him. Accompanying these forces is the secret of his chart.

What does the physician in charge write about him? All those specialists in and out of his "case", the nurses and other concerned parties? It is one thing to be told about lab and special procedure reports; it is very different to see those reports appended to progress notes. (One surprise was to see the medical student's admission note stating that this was the "first admission of an elderly male".)

Amidst this maelstrom of information, perhaps misinformation, the doctor/ patient's spouse and possibly children enter and exit the room. This adds to his discomfort since he is the object of pity.

Colleagues drop by to reassure him by quoting similar cases and their outcomes. He suspects that they are really reassuring themselves more than him. These physicians seem to mutter silently "there but for some reason go I. Glad I'm not in his bed." The doctor/ patient assiduously searches for their degree of care. Now he better comprehend what being a "case" entails. What probably constitutes efficiency by nurses, technicians and others is perceived as rather cold indifference. Longing for a soft or kind moment comes and goes episodically.

He begins to grasp what patients desire avidly - to know and to feel that they are in good hands. The venipuncturist could be swifter and target the vein more accurately rather than leaving his arm as a Kooning production in purple. He is aware of the many tentacles of the overruling Doctor-in-Charge, changing faces and figures that accompany the shift stops and rotations. He looks forward to the daily, hopefully b.i.d., visits of his caretaker physician. The resident, intern or (heaven forbid) medical student, who view him as only a humdrum or an interesting case, do not suffice. He would like to impress them, although his patient status reduces that likelihood, especially if he lacks a full knowledge of his own chart or case.

In some sort of extra-somatic fashion the doctor/ patient views himself as a medical Job, an innocent man whose weakness or defect has reduced him to the status of a patient. Patienthood is equated with punishment of the innocent by the omnipotent Doctor-in-Charge. Add to that posture and belief his position within a study, how does a placebo fit within the punishment scenario? Does it consist of more possible punishment, further tests or retribution?

Does he dare question the hands that care for him? Should he ask for a second opinion? Would that be oppositional behavior? Would he be questioning or defying the Doctor-in-Charge? What if the second opinion differs from the original diagnosis, where does the doctor/patient reside? With all these forces and vectors at work, can our doctor/ patient truly believe he is in good hands and accept his present diagnostic and treatment fate?

Denial would probably stand him in best stead in his perplexing posture of patienthood. The doctor could walk at an accelerated pace to his internist's office, state: "Can't be what it seems to be, because look, my overall body functions are good. Just do an EKG as a formality and then I'll go." Eventually I found some relief from my increasing concern about my fate. Denial persisted but at a lower intensity.

Eight years have elapsed since my bypass. I face further complications, less myocardial perfusion and left ventricular hypertrophy. Is this a slow progression to left ventricular failure? Despite a good ejection fraction, I harbor doubts, misgivings and anger at my devotion to science and a hit by a placebo. There is no glamour now - just regret. This cardiac-oriented world is forever with me. It permeates my nutrition, my athletic pursuits, my life. Every aspect of my life is balanced precariously on the slippery slope of my condition. There is a resurgence of self-directed anger when reflecting on the huge price paid for being "one of the group."

There is another aspect that emerges when surgery is completed and recovery commences. Depending on the immediate and long-term prognostication of results, the doctor/ patient faces some form of rehabilitation. He must confront the consequences in daily life. Do the findings and/ or results necessitate a change in life style? Has the narcissistic wound of patienthood healed over? Or has a residue accumulated? Will this denial mechanism return full-force, so that the physician will in effect resume previous patterns while disdaining the rehabilitative implications of his episode of illness.

In studies of bypass patients, most resumed within 6 months their previous (mostly Type A) behavior. Our doctor/ patient would most likely follow a similar gestalt of resurrection, slowly perhaps, of his way of physician patterns (doctoring doctrines?) of authority and independence; all proportional to his Medicare, Medicaid and managed care mentors!! Each phase of his resumption calls on his defense mechanisms to restore lifelong patterns of operation. I doubt that the doctor/ patient would extend these patterns, pressure himself to enter and to comply with a double-blind study. Placebo possibilities might well hint of deception and dependency.

In conjunction with writing this paper, I questioned a group of young to middle-aged psychiatrists as to their willingness to volunteer for a study similar to the Physicians Health Study. They unequivocally responded in the negative. The most verbal of the dissenters was a woman, who stated bluntly that she would never engage in an activity that was potentially dangerous to her. This in turn brought to the fore possible gender differences in response to placebo-involved studies.

The total picture reflects the doctor's traditional independence, power position and many of the above-described traits and his response to reversal of the doctor-patient relationship. The doctor struggles to become a patient and dislikes confronting the implications of a placebo involved study. Each of us debates the issues of ethics and responsibility. The personal resolution of these quandaries is critical to a physician's performance.

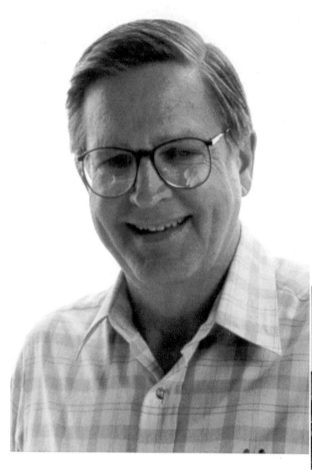
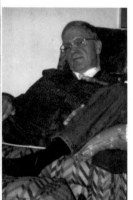

LIVING AND WORKING WITH LOU GEHRIG'S DISEASE

Edwin H. Church, M.D.

It is the summer of 1990 and I am sixty-five years old. I have been practicing psychiatry and psychoanalysis for thirty-five years.

I am starting my third year of the disease known as Amyotrophic Lateral Sclerosis (hereinafter referred to as "ALS") or more commonly known as Lou Gehrig's disease. It is a progressive wasting of skeletal muscles due to the death of motor nerve cells in the spinal cord. The cause is unknown. There is no treatment that arrests its progression. There is no cure.

My ALS began in the winter of 1987-88. I began to notice during my usual morning run that my left foot did not work well. This leg felt clumsy and seemed to hit the ground in an atypical fashion. Instinctively I felt that this should be checked with a neurologist, which I did in late March of 1988.

During the neurological examination I became concerned when the physician requested that I walk on my heels. I was incapable of doing this with either leg. The doctor indicated that I had some sort of peripheral nerve disorder and that he would perform a complete work-up to nail down the diagnosis. The work-up was completed in early May 1988.

Subsequent to the aforementioned work-up I went to a professional meeting in Montreal. Upon my return to New York I went to the neurologist for his final opinion. I still had no idea what was wrong, but I was constantly limping with my left leg. I never considered ALS as a potential cause of the limping, yet ALS was diagnosed to be "the cause". The electromyogram was evidently diagnostic and I was told that I had two to five years to live.

I was self-bombarded by questions for which I had no definitive answers: How fast would it progress? How do I want to spend my remaining years? Would I want to change anything that I was doing? How long will I be able to work? How would my wife and I survive if I reach a point where I can no longer earn any income? How would it feel to be like a helpless bowl of jello without any muscle power whatsoever? I had recently seen Dr. Stephen Hawking on a television program. He has ALS in a fairly advanced stage. He was almost unable to move any part of his body. His speech bordered on the incomprehensible. Would this be my fate? When would my breathing be affected? And my speech and swallowing? At this point I was still fairly strong. With the exception of the limp in my left leg, I was able to get around quite well. The extremes of ALS seemed far removed. Yet how far were they really?

Another big question was the future of my practice. Fortunately I had a fairly large practice. If my patients knew of my illness, would they want to drop me and switch to another therapist who enjoyed good health? One who would be more likely to be accessible throughout their treatment? What would my colleagues do when they discovered the nature of my illness? Would they stop referring patients to me? My decision - at that moment - was to tell no one. I eventually confided in a few close friends but saw no need to inform my patients until my problem became more obvious.

My neurologist suggested that I obtain a second opinion through an evaluation at Johns Hopkins Medical Center in Baltimore. Johns Hopkins was engaged in research on ALS and might have some kind of treatment available. Their evaluation confirmed my previous diagnosis. I did not qualify for their research program.

A colleague told me about a study being conducted at Mount Sinai Hospital in New York City. I applied and was accepted into this program as of January 1989. I was asked to take an experimental medication four times a day. The experimental medication consisted of three amino acids. I accepted the medication without any reluctance. I felt that it could do no harm and hopefully would effect some good. During a previous pilot study, the medication had been shown to slow or even stop the progression of ALS in some patients. I was, therefore, eager to give the medication a try. In addition to the medication, I spent one full day every three months at the ALS clinic at Mount Sinai Hospital. During each visit to Mount Sinai my blood was drawn and my breathing capacity was tested. I was also interviewed and examined by a neurologist and a psychiatrist, interviewed by a social worker and seen by an occupational therapist.

Course and Progression

The spread of muscle weakness leading to paralysis was in general quite slow. I soon began to realize that I would not die in the next few months, that I would be allowed time to adjust to the slowly progressive loss of muscle function. This loss of muscle function seemed to spread gradually from my feet to my legs, to my thighs, to my back, to my neck and most recently to my arms and hands. The main source of my dread was the cessation of the ability to swallow, to breathe and to speak. Every morning when I awoke I checked my breathing, expecting some sign of deterioration. More about this later.

I continued to maintain a busy schedule of private practice three days a week, seeing individual patients, groups and families. Two days a week I worked half-time at a busy outpatient psychiatric clinic affiliated with a large Bronx hospital. I found that the busier I was, the easier it was to forget for hours at a time that I was fatally ill. My leg weakness was reduced to a mere inconvenience by my demanding professional schedule.

After a routine clinic visit in February of 1989, it was suggested that I get prosthetic braces for my ankles and legs. The braces eliminated my foot drop and made walking firmer and easier. I went to a medical convention in Colorado in June of 1989 and did quite well. By the Fall of that year my balance, even assisted by the braces, was becoming unsteady and I required a cane. I could still manage without the cane if my walking was limited to the distance from my office to my waiting room and back. I hid the cane behind a drape in my office and hoped that my patients would not see me walking outside with the cane.

By the Fall of 1989, one cane was inadequate and a second cane was acquired in October, one cane for each hand. Walking half a city block had become quite arduous. My knees had become very unstable. The consequent risk of falling became a source of great apprehension. I fell several times , once stepping off the curb to hail a taxi and another time when turning a corner in the Bronx clinic. I fell stepping up to the curb and fell back into the path of oncoming traffic. Fortunately I was accompanied by several colleagues, who immediately took charge, redirected the traffic and obtained a wheelchair to convey me back to my office. On yet another occasion I fell while trying to get into the elevator of my residential building. I suddenly realized that there was no railing, nothing with which to pull myself upright. I crawled back to my apartment on my hands and knees and pulled myself up using the doorknob.

I reported at my next clinic visit, my series of falling incidents to my psychiatrist . He suggested that it was time to consider a walker or a wheelchair. My first real ride in a wheelchair was in March of 1990. I traveled by train for the funeral of a family member, which occurred in a town three hours away. A redcap wheeled me from the taxi to the train and another at the other end wheeled me from the train to the taxi. This same process occurred again later that year when I attended a family function in Boston. These experiences forced me to realize that I was disabled and that the disease would never go away. My image of myself had always been that of an athlete and of a physically strong person. This image began to change dramatically. Concurrently I was confronted by the issue of dependence, a matter with which I had limited experience. I had grown up an only child in a family that placed a high value on self-sufficiency and independence. The wheelchair brought home the fact that my dependency would steadily increase as the disease steadily progressed.

The Department of Physical Medicine offers a variety of wheelchairs. It dawned on me that there are excellent motorized wheelchairs and other types of vehicles available. This made my situation somewhat more tolerable, yet I felt strange. I attempted to become accustomed to my status one minute as a member of the patient population and then the next minute as a member of the physician population.

Telling the Patients

Once it became impossible to walk even a short distance without the use of both canes, it became clear to me that I must inform my patients about my illness. In general their reactions were similar. They typically responded with shock, surprise, sadness, even tears, and then compassion and support. Members of both my group therapies were very helpful. They met at my last appointment time of the day twice a week. Group members offered rides home, if they had a car, or offered to hail a taxi and assist me into it. Some patients expressed amazement that with such a life-threatening illness I could still listen to their complaints, which they perceived as comparatively trivial. Many inquired if I was in pain. I assured them that pain was not an integral part of my illness, unless I fell and injured myself. I also informed them that the disease affects only the musculature and does not negatively impact on one's thinking process or on one's mind. I stated that as long as my breathing and speech remained unimpaired, I would continue to work.

My fear that my patients would abandon me and find another therapist upon realizing I had Lou Gehrig's disease was fortunately never effectuated. Some patients expressed the opinion that if I had the courage to keep on working and to hang in there despite my illness, that they would stand by me. I told them that I could not be certain as to my continued availability for five years, or even for six months. All I could realistically relate to them was that my disease, according to my neurologist, would progress at the same rate as it had since its inception. Since initially my ALS had progressed at a slow rate, I had reason to assume that this would establish a pattern for the future.

Another issue that arose at this time was an ethical one. What should I say about my infirmity to new patients, who might require a long period of treatment? How much information was it fair to relay? If I spelled out my medical condition in a very detailed fashion, I could precipitate a substantial diminishing of my practice. I am over sixty-five; I could conceivably contract another illness that would prove fatal before the ALS did.

I finally came to the decision that I would assess each patient on an individual basis. I would advise the patient of my illness and explain the situation. To me this approach was fair. My infirmity was visible; I walked assisted by canes. Some patients seemed to pay little attention to my handicap and took it for granted that I required the canes. They were concerned with my ability to function as a psychiatrist, other considerations were superfluous.

I was also concerned that my patients would perceive me as too fragile and vulnerable, incapable of coping with assertive presentations of anger or other negative feelings. I did not want to hinder my patients' progress in therapy. This concern also proved to be groundless as my patients were not inhibited by my physical condition. Both my individual and group patients have freely expressed on occasion their anger.

My Own Reaction to the Illness

There seem to be hundreds of little changes that I have to adapt to as the disease progresses. For example, when I use the Automatic Teller Machine at my bank, I can insert the card but I now find it extremely difficult to coordinate my thumb and forefinger to remove the card. Some other individual must be called upon to assist me.

Zippers are difficult if not impossible to deal with. Light switches, turned on and off through manipulation of the thumb and forefinger, now require my use of pliers. Buttoning my shirt has become impossible.

Communication with other patients, met at the research project, and information gleaned from the project staff proved extremely useful. I learned that button hooks can be utilized and velcro patches can be substituted for shirt buttons. I appreciated the innovations yet I was angry. As the muscle weakness progressed and the weakness impacted directly on my hands and arms, I encountered numerous, seemingly endless areas of frustration which induced a great deal of anger. Simple everyday movements, once taken for granted, can no longer be performed easily if at all.

What about the fact that I have a disease that has killed everyone who has ever had it within a few years? I managed to start the grieving process, which I knew to be inevitable, while attending a professional meeting at a Gestalt workshop. Several months later I was able to get into a much more intensive grieving process with my wife and one of the nurses who attended me at that time. This provided a much-needed catharsis and a sense of relief.

Further Progression in Involvement of Breathing

I went along on a plateau for quite a while. During a professional meeting in the summer of 1990, I learned about the three-wheel electric cart, used by those who are incapable of walking. I purchased one in the fall of 1990 and utilizing it managed to attend meetings at

New York Hospital, where I had been on the voluntary attending staff for many years. I continued to get referrals and to work with my patients without difficulty. Only occasionally did questions about my illness arise. All in all I managed to retain fairly good spirits most of the time. I was visited frequently by friends, frequently called by them and maintained an active professional life. I began to collect video tapes of symphonies and concerts and began to study art history, because I had a collection of video tapes and an unread excellent textbook on the latter subject. I had considerable support from my family and my friends.

I began to get subtle hints that my breathing process was becoming impaired. The only prior subjective experience that I had was a little bit of asthma experienced daily and readily treated. I had already seen a pulmonary specialist and had several function studies done which indicated some breathing impairment. The specialist informed me that this had to be carefully monitored.

Late in January of 1991 I became aware that I was drifting off while attending patients. Some of my patients commented on this. I had no basis, however, to anticipate what occurred on February 5, 1991. I awoke as usual and discovered that I was too weak to get out of bed. My wife said that she would cancel that day's appointments and that I should stay in bed and rest. She looked in on me an hour later, found that my coloring was purple and gray and alarmed immediately dialed 911. The next thing I knew I was being treated on a cart by paramedics. The paramedics were doing endotracheal intubation which was providing me with oxygen. As I was only marginally conscious at this time, I did not experience any discomfort.

I was rushed to the emergency room of New York Hospital, which fortunately is only a minute from where I live. I spent the rest of the day in the emergency room, being examined, tested, x-rayed, etc. I was admitted to the Pulmonary Intensive Care Unit. There I was informed that I had been getting insufficient oxygen due to a weakness of my diaphragm. This condition could necessitate a tracheotomy and being placed on a respirator. I additionally learned that I had pneumonia, which was treated with medication. The tracheotomy was performed two days later. I had to become accustomed to life with a respirator and the plastic tubing connecting it to my trachea. I spent the next three weeks in the hospital. I improved to the point where I could return home with around-the-clock nursing and a portable respirator with which I had to learn co-existence.

Two weeks later I returned to the emergency room in acute respiratory distress. After extensive study it was ascertained that there was a blockage of one of my two principal bronchial tubes. This blockage was relieved through a bronchoscopy. I was readmitted to the hospital for a week, recovered promptly and returned home. During this interval my wife disposed of my professional office and of the family car.

Since this period of hospitalization, I have remained home. I spend most of my time connected to a respirator yet am still capable of being off it for intervals of two to three hours. My life consists of shuttling back and forth between the bedroom and the living room, which is the center of my social and professional life. It is in the living room that I read, watch television and see patients, friends and family.

In early May of 1991, I began meeting with one of my groups, which had continued to meet without me while I was hospitalized. This group now meets weekly in my living room. This arrangement seems to be working very well. Subsequent to the continuation of this group, I called some of my individual patients to inquire as to the resumption of their therapy. I see weekly about five or six people individually and a group consisting of eight people. My patients have rapidly become accustomed to my respirator and its somewhat funny noises. They completely overlook the respirator and concentrate on their therapeutic progress.

I plan to continue on this basis as long as possible. It is difficult to write prescriptions, but this limitation can be accommodated. Someone else can write them and I sign them, which I can still do. Fortunately my swallowing and speech have not been affected. Most importantly illness has not undermined, has not destroyed my ability to function effectively as a psychotherapist.

What does the future have in store? I have no idea. There is always hope that something new will be developed in the line of treatment. There was a recent genetic discovery regarding ALS, which holds promise that at some future time intervention with ALS can be done. I intend to keep living and working as long as I possibly can.

November 1992

My speaking has improved, although I am intubated and on a ventilating machine. The ventilating machine has a Passy-Muir Valve, which increases my ability to speak in conjunction with the machine. I am still continuing my practice. I see a group consisting of eight patients once a week and continue to see four patients individually. The money received through my practice precludes my receiving disability funds.

Though ALS has caused physical deterioration and concurrent physical restrictions, I am still mobile and, therefore, not confined to my residence. I can still move my arms though sometimes that movement is reduced to flailing. My area of activity has been expanded appreciably through my motorized chair and scooter. My scooter facilitates my travels from 74th to as far north as 86th Street, permits me to shop in my immediate neighborhood and allows me to go to weekly Grand Rounds at the Payne Whitney Clinic at New York Hospital.

There is a new experimental drug Regeneron which may be helpful. There has been a discovery that faulty glutamate metabolism may be damaging the neuronal transmission in ALS.

My wife is in a support group which has proven to be quite helpful. This group is conducted through the Manhattan Center for Living and led by a woman, who once a month commutes from Los Angeles to New York. I also have a support network, which includes among others an individual therapist and a person who cuts my hair and also administers Reiki Therapy.

Perhaps the greatest support that has evolved for me, I have realized internally. I have discovered a new interest in spirituality.

December 1997

Let us begin with my experience of life on the ventilator which has been the case for the past six years. What is it like to have ALS and live with the ever-present ventilator?

First of all it is rather precarious to say the least. The thing I have found most alarming is if the ventilator tube should come loose from its attachment to the tracheostomy tube at my neck - and it frequently does - there is no way I can call for help. This is because the tracheostomy site is below the vocal chords. In fact there are a number of places in the tubing system where interruptions occur and when they do I am without any air to breathe. For example there are three joints in the tubing before the tubing is one continuous tube all the way to the ventilator. Any of these can fall apart when subjected to the right amount of stress. This often occurs when I am being bathed and dressed during which I have to be turned several times. This is sufficient stress to cause any of the joints to fall apart. Of course the nurse is right there so she can reconnect the joint in a few seconds and no "air hunger" develops. Then there are two additional tubes which run next to the ventilator tube. They are much smaller in diameter and are called pressure tubes because they regulate the pressure in the system. They are attached to the system in such a way that they are separated fairly easily from their connection to the system and when that happens again I have no air to breathe.

Normally there is an alarm built into each ventilator which sounds to summon help. It goes off within ten seconds after any of these interruptions occur and usually brings help in a few moments. However, there was a time when I was in bed and my nurse was in the kitchen preparing my breakfast. She had set up a nebulizer treatment which means placing the nebulizer containing medication in line with my ventilator tubing and turning on the motor which drives the nebulizer. The tube simply fell from my neck meaning from that moment on I could get no air. But what I didn't know was that the alarm on the ventilator was not working! There was no way I could call for help! All I could do was watch my clock, worry and wait. I counted the eight minutes as they slowly passed and then I passed out. The next thing I remember was awakening in the ER at New York Hospital. My nurse looked very upset but was glad that I was regaining consciousness. She had brought my breakfast into the bedroom and found me unconscious, reconnected the tube and called 911. The ambulance came and took us to the ER. I realized after that experience how easily I could die.

When being transported from one room to another, my tubing is disconnected from the ventilator in the room I am leaving and reconnected to the ventilator in the room I am going to. On this occasion a nurse, taking me from the living room to the bedroom on the Hoya lift, could not find the on-off switch for the second ventilator in the bedroom. I could not tell her where that switch was. The entire trip lasts only thirty seconds, but in just thirty seconds I experienced air hunger. Finally she found the air switch but there was yet another problem. One of the pressure tubes had become disconnected and she did not know why the alarm was sounding. She looked everywhere, finally saw the loose tube and connected it.

There have been many other close calls but these two instances were the worst. I hope these incidents illustrate the next point I want to make about life on a ventilator and with ALS. It is the degree of dependency and utter helplessness to which I am now subjected. I was a person accustomed to considerable independence and self-sufficiency. It is very difficult to contend with a style of life that has been so dramatically altered, so irrevocably limited by illness.

Living dependent on a ventilator produces a condition not unlike chronic bronchitis. The air from the ventilator, although filtered, goes directly to the lungs bypassing the upper part of the respiratory system which does some filtration of its own. The air going directly to the lungs causes some irritation so various measures need to be taken to keep the bronchial system clear. These include nebulizer treatments two or three times daily usually followed by suction with a rubber catheter inserted into the trachea to pull the secretions out.

ALS is a disease in which there is a series of irreversible losses. First I lost the ability to stand and to walk, secondly the ability to breathe unassisted by machines and then the ability to use my arms and hands. The latter loss meant that I could no longer operate the joy stick on my electric wheelchair. My days of self-directed mobility were over. My nurse had to drive the wheelchair through use of a remote control device.

Finally I am losing the ability to speak comprehensibly. I am relying increasingly on a computer for communication. The computer is linked to a voice synthesizer which I can use to speak.

Considering all the losses which I have now experienced, the most difficult to accept was the loss of the use of my arms and hands. If I have an itch on my scalp or my ear there is nothing I can do about it. Friends who visit want to shake my hand but I can't lift my arm to meet their extended hand. My nurses have to feed me at mealtime. All my papers and files are handled by volunteers who come weekly to pay my bills and write my correspondence.

Another problem generated by my inability to use my arms and hand is a consequent inability to operate the remote for my television and VCR. This is a critical loss because television has become my window on the world. Because of my immobility it is almost exclusively television that keeps me apprised of life outside my apartment. As for my VCR I have been collecting videotapes of classical music both commercially produced and also recorded from TV broadcasts especially on PBS. I would estimate that I have 85 to 100 videotapes including music from Bach to Mozart to Beethoven to Brahms to Tchaikovsky and on into the twentieth century. I have three encyclopedias of music and musicology. This is how I spend much of my time. I must rely on my nurses to operate the remotes, put the cassettes into the VCR, operate the hifi system and keep track of the tapes.

Beginning in the Spring of 1996 I had a terrifying series of experiences. I was unable to get my epiglotis to shut. This meant that air would enter my trachea from the ventilator, bypass my lungs and go out my mouth. This was a rather alarming state of affairs. Air hunger would develop during a short time span. Initially this situation occurred after my pre-supper cocktail. The relationship between drinking an alcoholic beverage and the onset of the symptom became quite obvious so I had to give up all alcoholic beverages - one more loss to add to my collection. I discovered that if I drank water thus allowing myself something to swallow, the symptom would pass in ten or fifteen minutes. A few months later I was having waffles with syrup for breakfast. A similar side effect developed so I am now very careful about my consumption of sweets. Nowadays it will happen without any known precipitating factor but I learned from my pulmonary doctor that it can be treated by inflating the cuff or balloon on my tracheostomy tube.

I would like to stress that at no time has ALS caused me any physical pain. ALS is invariably fatal but with good nursing care and a few breaks it is bearable. I have been fortunate - a glaring exception occurred in 1994, which is unforgettable - in the forty or fifty nurses that I have had caring for me, who have been kind, competent and caring. In 1994 a new nurse had been assigned for the weekend. Sunday morning she came into my room and announced that she was going to punish me! I asked her what she was going to do. She replied that she was not going to bathe me, dress me or get me out of bed. I asked her to let me phone my family. She refused to let me make any phone calls. I consequently spent the day in bed, from where she allowed me to watch television. It was after that experience that I found an emergency call service which I could call easily by pressing a button. I called this nurse's agency the next day and told her supervisor what had happened. The supervisor told me the nurse would be removed from duty and required to get treatment.

December 1998

Very little has changed during the last year. My speech is gone due to the loss of muscles in the throat and mouth which enables us to form words. The computer does my speaking. When I don't have access to the computer, i.e. in the bedroom while being bathed and dressed, I have an alphabet board which has all the letters on it . The nurse points to each line systematically and when she gets to the line my letter is on, I blink. The nurse then goes across the indicated line until she reaches the letter that I require to compose a message. This is a very slow process but it is quite effective. I gradually learned more short cuts which expedited this method of communication.

Life continues but continues with a variety of problems to contend with. I spent the last week of June in the hospital with intestinal obstruction. This was diagnosed as paralytic ileus, which is functional and not organic. It was somehow related to a urinary tract infection. Antibiotics and one pint of magnesium citrate took care of the intestinal obstruction.

My teeth have become my enemy. Because of the loss of muscles in my face, under certain conditions (i.e. when being suctioned my jaw undergoes convulsive movements) I bite my tongue, cheeks and lower lip. These are reflexive actions which I can't control. All I can do is keep my jaws locked together as tightly as possible. This, however, does not completely preclude the biting. ALS has also affected my eyelids. By evening I have to struggle to keep my eyes open, especially the right eye. My epiglotis continues to pose an area of difficulty as it becomes increasingly flabby. Air comes in from my ventilator and exits the glotis, thereby bypassing my lungs. There are two tiny balloons attached to the trach tube accessible by means of a slender plastic tube which dangles from my neck. By inflating the balloons the pressure in my larynx increases, forcing air into my lungs. This allows me control over this process.

My routine hasn't changed over the past year. How do my days go by? My day begins at 9 AM because my schedule is determined by that of the nurses who have a 12-hour shift beginning at 8 AM. First I have my vital signs taken and then I get tracheostomy care and suctioning of my trachea. Trach-care means changing the gauze around the tracheostomy tube and cleaning the tracheostomy site with peroxide and saline solution and then putting fresh gauze on. Suctioning means putting a rubber catheter hooked to a machine which provides suction down into my trachea from the tracheostomy site and suctioning out any secretions which have accumulated and which might compromise breathing. The bandage around my gastrostomy tube also has to be changed twice daily. Then I get a shave and a bath in bed. After that I get dressed, rolled onto the canvas sling of the Hoya life and wheeled out to the living room and placed in my recliner chair where I usually spend the rest of the day until 11 PM when I go to bed.

I spend time in a variety of ways. The nurse who helps me with my morning routine usually wants to have lunch between 12 and 1 o'clock. While the nurse is eating, I either watch TV or have her set up the computer so that I can write. After the nurse has finished lunch we make some phone calls and once a week she takes me out in my electric wheelchair around the neighborhood. There are a number of places we can go. We nearly always go to the supermarket and pharmacy and sometimes to the bank, card shop, stationery store, book store or hardware store. Occasionally we go to New York Hospital, only four blocks south of my apartment building, where most of my doctors have their offices. My internist who runs my case makes house calls every Thursday, visiting every other week.

In retrospect this has been a good year. I've started to write a book about the challenges of coping with ALS. My nursing care has continued to be excellent. Friends come to call frequently especially since I live near New York Hospital and many of them are on the staff there. My New Jersey family visits now and then, my Arizona family visits once a year. So, in spite of being quadriplegic, unable to breathe on my own, unable to speak or enjoy the taste of food, I am glad to be alive.

Editor's Note:

Dr. Church passed away on April 16, 1999. He had been admitted to the hospital on April 14, 1999 for observation of suspected pneumonia. During the night, Dr. Church went into cardiac arrest and wasn't resuscitated for over 12 minutes leaving him in a comatose state with little chance of recovery. Dr. Church had a living will that instructed that if he became comatose and obviously wasn't going to recover, all life support equipment and measures be discontinued. His family carried out his instruction on April 16, 1999. Dr. Church died at 6:30 PM.

On May 22, 1999 a memorial service was held for Dr. Church in New York City. Family, colleagues, friends and former patients honored his memory with accolades attesting to his unwavering dedication to live life to the fullest in spite of any obstacles that came his way. In the 12 years that he suffered from this affliction, he never complained about his circumstances. He was a courageous man. Dr. Church was a devoted classical music lover. His ashes were scattered over the lawn at Tanglewood music center in Massachusetts. His two sons, their wives and two grandchildren survive him. (Dr. Church's family provided this information.)

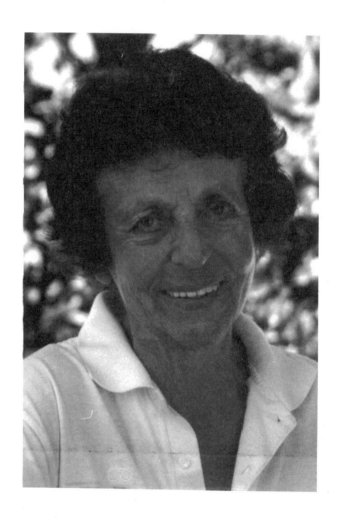

Judita Hruza, M.D.

SURVIVING THE HOLOCAUST

Judita Hruza, M.D.

This writing is about the Holocaust. It is
not intended as a documentary, although
the dates are all correct and the events
accurate. My intention is to reveal my
perceptions of these events, to convey my
reactions to varied experiences and to
attempt to identify those factors, which
proved pivotal to my survival.

I came from a middle class Jewish family, from a
little village in Czechoslovakia on the Hungarian
border. When part of Czechoslovakia including my
village was added to Hungary in 1938 (Hitler's gift to the
loyal Hungarians), we found ourselves in an entirely different world. Life in prewar Czechoslovakia was fair and
free. There was no official anti-Semitism. In our new home-
land in Hungary, we found ourselves to be objects of national attention, an additional burden for Hungary. The
government had to amend the existing anti-Jewish laws,

regulating Jewish participation in every facet of Hungarian life. There were restrictions for schools, public jobs, businesses, etc. I could not plan to be educated beyond high school. My family's economic existence became uncertain.

On the other side of the border in the new Slovak State, the anti-Jewish laws went far beyond the Hungarian restrictions. President Tess, the leader of the Catholic Slovak party, bragged that his laws were even stricter than the German rulings. My grandparents' and my uncle's belongings were seized. They were moved out of their houses and in 1942 deported to a "death camp" in Poland, Auschwitz. The Shadow of the Holocaust fell on my family long before my immediate family was directly affected.

A letter written by my grandmother to my mother was smuggled out of the death camp. It contained horrible descriptions of her ordeal. My mother cried for days after receiving the letter. My grandmother told us that my 82 year old grandpa had died in a crowded freight car. My grandma felt that she would soon be selected to die. I didn't want to hear any more details and I ran from the house sobbing. When I returned I asked that my mother never show me the letter and never discuss its contents with me. I felt I would die if I heard of more horrors affecting my adored grandparents. My mother never again mentioned my grandparents, except to relate that her parents would be happy to know that we were still safe and together. My grandparents wouldn't want their grandchildren's precious years to be spoiled by worrying and mourning. My grandmother would say "You'll know when you have your own children."

My parents tried to make my brother's and my own life as good as was possible. They wanted us to be well educated, to read, to learn foreign languages, to prepare for life after the war. My mother instilled in us a very strong belief that life is precious. As long as one is alive, things can change for the better and it is always worth it to hold out as long as possible. She had a unique ability to find something good in every situation. Although slim, fragile in appearance and readily moved to tears, she was clear headed and efficient in emergencies. My mother was a tower of strength. I could come to her with every trouble, pain or confusion and she would comfort me, make me feel safe, loved and hopeful. She had an enormous capacity for extending comfort and many people sought her out for this reason.

Between 1938 and 1944, we lived the very restricted lives of Hungarian Jews. My father began to wear black ties to symbolize his mourning for the Jewish people. We lived in constant worry and with the ever present awareness of impending doom. However, we were still safe and survived with hope. As the war progressed, the Germans increasingly lost battles. It seemed realistic that we could survive until the end of the war, the anticipated Allied victory. This illusion came to an end on March 19, 1944. Germany occupied Hungary.

My brother and I lived and went to school in Budapest. Two hours after hearing of the German occupation, we went to the train station. We were denied access to the trains - we were Jews. We were shocked, in grief beyond endurance. Our sole aspiration was to be reunited with our parents. We exchanged letters full of anguish, love and hope. The letters conveyed encouragement and promises of survival and reunion. We never saw our parents again. They were deported to Auschwitz in May 1944. Two and a half months after the German occupation, the countryside was cleared of its entire Jewish population.

My brother and I stayed with our family's Jewish friends. We lived, one family per room, in one of the assigned yellow-starred houses. There were air raids twice a day accompanied by severe bombing. Most of us were not very fearful of the bombing. The possibility of death by the German or Hungarian Nazis posed a far greater danger than did the bombs. We felt a certain satisfaction at the prospect of German and Hungarian military installations being annihilated, of Hungarian Nazis cowering in their shelters.

When Ferenz Szalasi the leader of the Hungarian Nazi Party assumed power in October of 1944, the Jews of Budapest were deported. At this time, the Russian army had already crossed the Hungarian border. Trains were required exclusively for military use. The government consequently found another, inexpensive way to move on foot thousands of people. It began with an announcement ordering every man age 16-60 and every woman 16-40 to report to work at a sports stadium. We were to bring warm clothes, strong shoes and a 3-day food supply. As we started the march, the huge crowd of young women resembled a summer camp gathering. I felt strong, tough and capable of enduring any hardship.

My awakening occurred on the first night. We had to walk for several hours to reach our destination, an airport. A steady rain soaked the clothes on our backs and the contents of our canvas backpacks, multiplying the weight of those items. The heavy mud on our shoes made each step an extra burden. In vain we asked for rest. We consoled ourselves with the vision of a dry and warm place at the airport. We arrived at the airport late at night and were literally pushed through the gate. We walked up some stairs in the dark and pouring rain. We were pressed together tightly, still in the rain. The airport had no roof. We spent the evening standing in icy rainwater which reached to our knees. In the morning as the room was emptied, some women collapsed. These were the first victims of the deportation. They had died during the night and "dropped dead" when the support of other bodies was removed. This experience foreshadowed other and worse experiences. The goal of our captors became clear to us. They didn't want us to work; they wanted us to die.

The march continued the next day. First we were herded eastward to dig anti-tank trenches against the Russian Army. When the front approached, we were directed back toward Budapest. We expected (hoped) to be returned home but this never happened. Instead we were brought to a large brick factory. The factory had a roof but no walls so we were subject to an incessant November wind. We should have been grateful for that roof. This was the last time for over a week that we slept under a roof. We wandered through western Hungary for 12 days. Our accommodations during that period were very imaginative: a soccer field, a village square, the belly of a freighter (the guards were spreading rumors about sinking unwanted cargo), a hay market, pigsties still warm from the pigs, a freshly plowed field and a barn where the loft collapsed killing many prisoners.

Our final destination was Koszeg, a Hungarian town on the Austrian border. This was one of eight camps, whose prisoners dug anti-tank trenches to protect Austria from the advancing Russian army. The Russians reached the Austrian border in March of 1945 and the Germans retreated into Austria. The camps were evacuated. The sick and weak prisoners were killed while the ambulatory were marched to Mauthausen in Upper Austria. This march lasted 17 days, March 28-April 15, 1945. It was hard to tell how many of our original group had survived since we were joined by several other groups. It has been calculated that, during the month of April 1945, 80,000 to 100,000 Hungarian Jews were involved in the death marches. In Mauthausen and Gunskirchen about 40,000 Jews were liberated. I don't know how many Jews died after liberation.

Mauthausen was evacuated after 10 days. We were directed toward Gunskirchen, a camp almost totally unknown to the public but yet another symbol of German arrogance. This camp was constructed in March of 1945, 6 weeks before the Unconditional Capitulation.

The Gunskirchen camp was located in a dense and swampy pine forest. There were eight barracks to house 17,000 people. There was no straw, latrines, bunks or water except that dripping from the trees. We lay on top of each other. We survived on one cup of soup a day. There was no bread. This was the camp where the flesh of dead prisoners was carved out and eaten. On May 4, 1945 Gunskirchen was liberated by the US Army and my perception of this camp changed radically. This was a glorious camp!

Surviving Against Deadly Odds

Whenever I relate my Holocaust experience I am repeatedly asked the same question. How did you manage to survive all the horrors, the starvation, the lice, the selections, the shootings while so many perished? The odds were against me. Death came in so many forms and so frequently that an individual's chance of survival was negligible. In Gunskirchen Death Camp prisoners died at a minimum rate of 200 a day. If the US Army had arrived six weeks after its actual liberation date, they wouldn't have found a single survivor.

I searched my mind to solve a puzzle that has always been a mystery to me. What helped me to survive? During my childhood and early adolescence I was considered to have "delicate" health, to be fragile, thin and sickly. During school hiking trips I was left at home. The teachers thought that I was incapable of maintaining the pace of my peers. When I returned to Budapest after the war, a former classmate was surprised to see me. She thought I would have been among the first victims of the Holocaust.

Prior to deportation my general attitude and mental state were dominated by fear and at times by panic. I was terrified of death, of pain, of the SS and every form of violence. I considered suicide though suicide was contingent on the discovery of an easy, painless way to do it. Ultimately I discovered that though living in close proximity to death I wanted to survive. I had never realized with what tremendous force this will for survival existed in me. I experienced a level of anger that I thought myself incapable of sustaining. I did not want to make the Germans' job easier for them by dying. I discovered in myself an unquenchable love of life that had been instilled by my mother. I had a strong faith that my parents and my brother would survive because they would do everything within their power to survive. I felt an obligation to survive so I could be reunited with my family. I was also curious, very curious about starting life from scratch. I couldn't imagine life without anti-Jewish laws.

I was extremely fortunate throughout the death marches and the death camps. I was not alone. My mother's best friend Anna, my surrogate mother in Budapest, had to report for "work" with me. She also was a member of the designated age group for women, 16-40 years old. Anna was very practical in hardship situations and very supportive when my spirits lagged. During the 3 or 4 AM Apell (head count), I used to cry in the bitter cold. My frostbitten toes hurt in my boots. Aunt Anna used to comfort me: "Don't cry, baby. When we get home, I'll make hot chocolate for you and serve you breakfast in bed." On our way to digging the anti-tank trenches, we spotted a little dog running out of a farm. It reminded me of Anna's 12-year old son. I pointed out this resemblance to Anna. Both the dog and Anna's son were well and cheerful. After this exchange we looked forward to encountering the little dog.

The two of us established a few principles to observe in critical situations: never volunteer for light work, refuse a ride in favor of walking, never mention personal illness and never be taken to the hospital, from which there was no departure. We believed that we had a better chance of survival if we exhibited usefulness by doing the heavy work and carrying the heavy loads.

One day two trucks drove into our camp. The guards announced that women, too weak for digging, could work in a factory. Women with poor feet and poor shoes should also report for this indoor job. Many women eagerly climbed on the trucks, which filled rapidly. An SS-man surveyed the rest of us. "You two, get on the truck". I stopped in front of the man, pointed to our hiking boots and replied in perfect German: "Our shoes are fine. We are strong. We don't need light work!" The SS-man looked at our feet and waved his hand: "Na gut (all right), stay!" The trucks drove away. We learned from the returning guards that the women were taken to Auschwitz.

On another occasion, I was diagnosed by a fellow prisoner, an M.D., to have appendicitis. He advised: "You should report sick, stay home and put a cold compress on your stomach." I was more afraid of the "sick status" than of a burst appendix. I went to work and pretended to work, although exertion was inevitable and my performance poor. I did not contract peritonitis nor was I shot. I had avoided certain death in the sick tent, where patients were locked in and deprived of food and water. The sick tents opened only to take new patients in and move the dead ones out. Nobody left these tents alive. My appendix did not bother me again until I was safely back in Budapest. There it was removed, just prior to perforation.

As time dragged on, everyone developed some kind of "street smart" (or rather "camp smart") tricks to cheat death. I considered almost everything that grew to be edible - grass, leaves, potato peels, bread mold, slops. My eating habits were inclusive of few limits; I could not force myself to eat live snails as others did nor could I resort to cannibalism. Another rule of survival was - always keep a piece of bread until you get another one. I was able to adhere to this rule for a period of 5 days. On the fifth day, no new food arrived. I felt I would die if I continued starving and I began to panic. I imagined myself lying dead of starvation with a slice of uneaten bread in my bag. I ate the bread.

To keep from freezing to death, we soon discovered the solution - body heat. Sleeping outdoors you had to lie between two other prisoners, pressed together. People lying at the end positions were often found dead in the morning. We finally solved this problem by forming a circle. This unfortunately was only possible where the ground was flat , otherwise people had to lie with their heads lower than their feet.

While in the camps, killing lice was critical. Each night after work we spent hours inspecting the seams of our clothes, killing one by one the lice and nits. It developed into a game. We competed for the highest number killed. That number was in the hundreds. The little beasts multiplied at an extraordinary rate. If you skipped a single night of inspection, the numbers had doubled by the following day. If you skipped two nights, you had no strength to get up because of the loss of blood. We had a term for the self-destructive behavior of those who ignored the lice: "He laid himself down on the straw." This meant that he had given up. This person stopped going to work, consequently received a half-food ration and died within 3 to 5 days. During the Death Marches you required more willpower to stay alive. You had to keep in step, never lag behind, never stop or sit down. Any of these actions could result in death. I had to remind myself constantly that I had to be the last one to give up. As long as hundreds were still able to walk, I would walk.

In addition to these acquired tips for survival, my mind developed several tricks of its own to protect me from giving up. After my unsuccessful attempt to escape in Budapest, returned to the deportation group - beaten, hopeless, sore and soaked, marching over the Danube bridge toward Germany, I experienced a strange sensation. Many years later, while attending medical school, I identified this feeling as "depersonalization". During the march I felt separated from my body, my feelings, my very being. I felt as if I had nothing in common with the girl who marched among thousands in the rain. I floated in the air and looked down at the sad downtrodden crowd which dragged itself toward its ominous destination. I felt compassion for this mass of humanity, but I didn't feel their pain or even my own pain. It wasn't until we were ushered into a sheltered brewery cellar, that I became aware of myself.

At 3 A.M. while on our way to the West we were subjected to a robbery. The perpetrator was the least likely person in the least likely place. A man, attired in the garb of a Catholic priest and accompanied by two dignified, elderly women, ordered us to line up in the churchyard. All three had large crosses around their necks. The priest also wore an arrowcross armband (the Hungarian Swastika) and had a gun on his shoulder. He ordered us to surrender all our money, jewelry, arms (including pocketknives), pens and pencils and to drop them in the two ladies' laundry baskets. I put my money in the basket but retained my watch, a birthday present from my parents.

When they finished accumulating our possessions, the priest made a speech: "this is your donation for the soldiers on the frontier, Now I'll show you what happens to the thieves who cheat and try to hide some valuables." Another man wheeled a wheelbarrow towards us. In the wheelbarrow was a dead body. The corpse's face had been beaten to a pulp. The priest then told us to drop in the baskets anything that we had not previously relinquished. Frightened I gave up my precious watch. The women then offered us drinking water - "to show you we are merciful." We were then permitted to continue our march.

During the long march from Budapest to the Austrian border, our misery grew by the mile. We received food every three days. We drank from puddles in the road. The incessant rain ran down our backs. The backpacks seemed to weigh a ton. Everyone acquired dysentery. If you stopped for relief you received a blow to the head or you were shot. We kept walking, our body fluids and blood running down our legs. Our rows did not resemble those of an organized march. We were ghosts and shadows in rags. We moved slowly. We left clothing, bags, dead bodies and even children's toys behind.

One day an important event occurred. A diplomatic car with a tiny Swedish flag pulled over to our rows. A young man (now I know it was Raol Wallenberg) got out and handed us a canvas sack full of papers. He said in German, "My friends, distribute these "Schutzpasses" among yourselves. Use them as you can. Good luck!" These documents were passports declaring that the bearer was placed under the protection of the Swedish government and could not be deported. In Budapest there were special buildings assigned to house these chosen citizens. We did as we had been told. Anna and I had received 2 mother-daughter passes with strangers' names but similar ages. A new energy came into us. We were the fortunate owners of passports to life! We could hardly wait to present our new passports to the authorities. The last few days on the border seemed much easier. We almost forgot the dysentery epidemic, the sore feet and the constant November rain. I fantasized about a hot bath and a bed with clean sheets in a sheltered house under the royal protection.

Finally the owners of these precious papers were standing in line facing the uniformed six-man committee. All six wore arrowcross armbands, the insignia of the Hungarian Nazi party. We saw trucks with Red Cross signs, waiting to take us back to safety. I experienced palpitations and was shaking when I handed our papers to them and waited for them to be examined. A wall of bricks crashed down on me! They tore both passes into shreds, saying, "These are not valid. They were issued after October 15." It was all over. The Red Cross trucks departed with a few lucky passengers. The rest of us marched toward the dreaded border. At first I was in shock. I moved automatically in a daze with the crowd. Then I realized the import of this occurrence, we were leaving the country and we were destined for destruction.

Does it make any sense to fight, to put so much painful effort into step after step, which will only bring us closer to inevitable death? Why not just sit down on the roadside, accept a shot and be free from all the pain? I was looking for a spot to rest when for the first time in my life, I heard a voice. I did not know then about hallucinations. I was convinced that it was my mother talking to me. She said, "My poor little heart, don't give up. When you talk to your children and friends, this horrible ordeal will be just an episode in your life when you are twenty". I didn't know then that my mother was dead. She had been killed six months earlier in Auschwitz. After I heard the voice I calmed down. My mother had never lied to me. I became almost elated. I told Anna not to worry that "We'll be all right". I treasured this experience and re-played the message in my mind every time I was confronted by a particularly low point.

As time passed, my state of mind gradually changed. I evolved into a different person through this process. I lost the human values that I had been taught while growing up in a decent, loving, cultured family. After 3 to 4 months of camp life, there were very few rules of decency, morality or civilization that I wouldn't break (at least in my mind) to sur-vive. My self-imposed limits were few - not to steal from a fellow prisoner and not to eat human flesh. I had no second thoughts about stealing apples from a roadside shed, squat-ting and relieving myself or taking a blanket from a corpse. During the months of deportation I became so accustomed to the scenery and the hardship of daily life that I became oblivious to the smell of burning old clothes, the sight of dead bodies scattered everywhere and the faces of live prisoners, similar in appearance to the skulls of skeletons. The smells and the sights were reduced to inconsequential background.

These sensations evoked no more emotion than I experience today pushing my cart through a supermarket. On rare occasions I was aware that I had reduced the horrific to the prosaic and that another world did still exist. This insight occurred only when I got a glimpse of that other world.

It was Easter Sunday and the sun was rising. We were wet, muddy, filthy as we held our steaming blankets over smoking, dying little campfires. I saw a girl on a bicycle. She was about my age and she was strikingly clean. Her shiny long hair, crisp white dress, polished shoes, sparkling bicycle, the flowers in her basket - everything looked freshly scrubbed, fragrant and radiant. I became intensely aware of the army of lice that crawled across my skin. She glanced at me with a look of horror. At that moment one idea consumed me - in another life I had looked like this girl!

Another pivotal memory concerns a fellow prisoner. During our rest at the roadside, she was given a bowl of rice by a German soldier. I watched her spoon travel between the bowl and her mouth. I fantasized that she dropped dead and I ate the rest of her rice. I watched the remnants of rice disappear into her mouth and despaired because the girl lived and the rice was gone.

During an air raid, Mauthausen camp was bombed. We were ordered out of our tents and we watched the fireworks in the great outdoors. I saw body parts and whole bodies fly through the air. There were explosions, fire and screams. The earth shook beneath us. My only worry was that the building housing the food should survive the bombardment.

In Mauthausen we lived in huge tents intended for 200 occupants but used by six times that number. There was no work, no water, no straw, no latrines, no Appells. There were two daily routines, morning inspection and food. The inspection was performed by an SS-man wielding a club, who walked through narrow aisles and randomly struck prisoners on the head. The food was brought by the kapos (Kamarad Polizei), who were usually Polish prisoners. Six year veterans of death camp life, the survivors of hell, they had become ruthless and cruel. They brought us soup after first removing the solid parts, the potatoes and vegetables. We survived on the residue, the salty water. They brought only half of the bread, one loaf per twenty people rather than one loaf per ten. What they pilfered, the kapos traded for cigarettes and services from prisoners located outside the camp (non-Jewish prisoners, housed in wooden barracks with electricity and water - the "palace").

Our daily sustenance arrived at any time of the day. Our only activity was to watch the camp entrance and wait for that glorious moment. I tried to force myself to THINK. Some people talked incessantly of food while others screamed in vain at them to stop. Men and women recited recipes in great detail. This disturbed me because I could not recall the elegant, delicious dishes only the bread, potatoes, milk and apples. I wondered why I had never eaten raw potato peels with salt, a delicacy in the camp. I tried to occupy my mind with thoughts other than food. This proved impossible. I was unable to recall a single rhyme or tune, to remember the plot of a book, a movie or a play. In my mind I searched for my mother so I could complain to her but I couldn't see her face. I did not remember what she looked like! I tried desperately to envision my home and my family but the picture was reduced to my mother's hand dishing out soup into my bowl. I could readily conceptualize each piece of meat, vegetable and noodle. I could see the soup's rising steam but I could not see the faces of my family around the table.

Our meal finally arrived. It was grayish, dirty water clouded with a few grains of farina. It was served lukewarm. My only complaint was that there was so little of it, just half a bowl. The bread was marbled with bright green mold - good news. There were still finicky people who picked out the mold to discard it. I begged them for the green crumbs. Sometimes I collected a cupful of this green delicacy. Anna and I ate it slowly, savoring every bit of it. Our delicacy was probably a lifesaver. It provided not just additional calories but probably penicillin.

During the long winter of 1944/45 we stayed in one place, a camp on the Hungarian side of the Austrian border near the little town of Koszeg. We stayed there for four months. We ineffectively dug anti-tank trenches in frozen ground. The Germans must have concluded that women were useless for this job and consequently arranged frequent "selections for light work". Those selected were shipped directly to Auschwitz, a fact unknown to us then. The remaining women occupied only 2 of the 50 cardboard tents in the camp. The other 48 were for men. The tents were set up in rows. After dark no one could leave the tents except to use the latrines. The prisoners had to call out to the guards, "Guard, small bathroom (No. 1) or big bathroom (No. 2)." This meant that you stepped out next to your tent or went to the far-away latrine.

I am still amazed by the courage and dedication of one newsman K. Havas Geza, who defied the curfew making his daily rounds with the news of the war front. His hands were crippled by frostbite. He couldn't open doors; he could only knock. He stood within each tent for a minute and reported the latest position of the retreating German army. Everyone excitedly anticipated his visit. It was the highlight of the day. He brought us hope, the chief ingredient in the recipe for survival. In rain, snow, ice and wind, he never missed his visits. Each day, when he stepped out of his tent without alerting a guard, he put his life in mortal danger. He survived the night walks but was later killed during the Eisenerz massacre on April 7, 1945.

On Saturday, April 7, 1945 - the 10th day of the Death March, we received a hearty meal of bread and soup. We then climbed a steep road into the mountains. As we got closer to the top, we heard louder and louder shots. The road continued downward and beyond a bend we saw the guards on both sides of the road. Their guns trained on us; they shot into our rows. The road was littered with dead and wounded bodies. Bags, clothes and mud were shiny and red from blood. The guards yelled, "rush, rush Jewish pigs!". The guards were everywhere, on both sides and in front of us. We all understood what was happening; the Russian and American armies were close. Stuck between these two advancing fronts, we were a burden to the Germans. There was no need for us. There was no work, no food, no shelter. This was a deserted place with no witnesses and no route of escape. The food in the camp was the fuel to carry us to our execution.

This was clear to all of us but we were governed by an animal's instinct for survival. Why did nobody try to run off the road on the steep slope? Or just sit down instead of jumping over the bodies, stumbling and slipping? Instead we kept running en masse, pressed tightly together, anxious not to draw attention to ourselves. It was snowing slightly and suddenly for a few seconds the sun appeared. There was a collective audible sigh. I thought as did others - the sun is shining but not for me! People around me dropped like flies. Some screamed; others prayed aloud. I screamed, "Mommy, don't let them do this!" I thought of the piece of bread that I had saved in vain. I promised that "I'll be good, I'll be so good!" I thought of the sea that I would never see. I realized that I did not know how to die; it was a test for which I had not prepared. Suddenly I just wanted enough time to take twenty breaths. I thought of the zillions of breaths that I had taken - without a thought - during the last twenty years. Now I begged for just twenty more breaths. The shooting lasted for 40 minutes. 500 people were killed; 200 survived.

The remaining prisoners were ordered to stop, to stand at attention, not to move, not to talk. The guards walked around us, saying, "It's not dark yet." There was no more shooting. Taking a great risk, I secretly fished out my bread and ate it crumb by crumb. Two hours later we marched into a camp with barracks. I whispered to Anna, "Do you think they'll let us live?"

Let me jump ahead by 20 years. I revisited this spot with my children, ages 8 and 13. I recognized the scenery, the tall pine trees and the snow-covered mountaintops. I searched for some sign, some memorial to the 500 killed here. There was no memorial - only a poster announcing an upcoming circus. In the valley we purchased postcards of Eisenerz. A friendly shopkeeper inquired whether this was our first trip to this picturesque area. I told him about my previous visit. He nodded gravely and said," Yes, I remember it. The prisoners were fed on the bottom of the hill." I told him what happened on our way to the valley. No longer friendly, his face turned from pink to deep red, "This is a damn lie! Nobody was killed here. Maybe one or two of them tried to run away. Maybe in Mauthausen. But never in Eisenerz. Don't do communistic propaganda in my shop!" I charged toward the shopkeeper. If my brother hadn't stopped me I would have killed the store owner with my bare hands. My brother half carried me out, comforting me, "He is not worth it. Come, don't even look at him." I understood now why there was no memorial to be found.

This story came to a better ending in the spring of 1993. I participated in a documentary movie about the Death Marches in Austria, made by a talented producer Michael Zuzanek. Again I stood on the same mountain. There were no guns directed at me, only a camera. I had the opportunity to tell the story of the Eisenerz massacre for the whole world to hear. As a result of the film "Alle schweigen" (All be silent) memorial monuments were raised at several locations in Austria. There was finally a monument in Eisenerz to commemorate my admired newsman and the 500 who died with him.

Another hero of Koszeg was a young physician, whom everybody called Laci. One frosty morning the guards were chasing people out for "Appel". Laci had set up a makeshift operation table in his tent and was amputating the gangrenous leg of a fellow prisoner. The guard ordered him out for "Appel". He answered, "I can't stop now. He is bleeding too much." The guard said playfully, "I give you a choice. You go to Appel now and I let you live or you can finish surgery and I shoot you." The doctor didn't even look up. He finished his work and dressed the wound. The guard watched him patiently. When Laci was done, the guard raised his gun and shot him in the head.

This incident confirmed my belief that physicians share a secret that renders them strong, invincible and fearless. During the Death Marches when we arrived at our nightly camps, us common folk looked for the best place to sleep, collected firewood to dry our soaked blankets or just sat and rested our aching feet. The doctors, who had endured the same painful march as we had, set up makeshift tents with a Red Cross sign that offered treatment on demand. The doctors had to carry their medical bags in addition to their personal belongings. Where did they get the extra energy and motivation to place their patients' needs above their own? I decided that if I survived, I would become a doctor. At that time the probability of survival was almost zero so I was not preoccupied with my future profession. My thoughts were centered on the more mundane - survival, one painful hour at a time.

I will jump ahead in my story once again. I arrived home in Budapest in August 1945. My 16 year old brother was alive but our parents, grandparents and other relatives were dead. We had no home, no property and no money. My brother was a high school student. I looked for a job to support us. One day my brother presented me with a medical student registration card in my name. He had enrolled me secretly. He said, "Everybody can be admitted now, Jewish or not. You would be a fool, not to study. Don't worry, we'll make it." Five years later I graduated as an M.D.

The day of our liberation started as any other day. The SS-men were marching between the barracks, knocking down anyone who got in their way. The noise of the far away explosions sounded nearer. The SS suddenly ordered everyone into the barracks. Rumors began to spread that the SS were leaving the camp. Somebody saw a white sheet at the main building. One by one we sneaked out of the barracks. There were no guards. We didn't know what to do. Most of the prisoners remained lying on the floor, too weak to move. Some were seized by a feverish activity; they sought the SS. Others broke into the food store. There were those who just went crazy - dancing, singing, cuddling imaginary babies in their arms.

Anna spoke of the future but I was incapable of absorbing what she was saying. For me freedom had become frightening. I had no idea how to do anything without an order. Where would I get food if not given my 4 oz. ration of bread? How would I get home? What will I find at home? Who will I find alive? This should have been the happiest day of my life. I had won - I lived, but I had forgotten how to be happy.

The next morning everyone capable of walking went to meet our liberators. The walk through the unguarded gate seemed unreal. The dirt road toward the highway was littered with dead bodies, lying on their stomachs in a crawling position. They had died on their way to freedom. We finally saw the colony of US jeeps. The soldiers waved the V-signs and threw packs of cigarettes and candy bars at us. Our ghost-like appearances were reflected in their horrified eyes when they looked at us.

A new nightmare started. A few hours later we found an open German Army storehouse. Hundreds of starved, half-crazed people invaded a huge hall, full of canned food, sugar, macaroni. Some dug their heads into the sugar until they suffocated. Others pushed more and more food into their mouths, gagged, choked, doubled up in pain and died. The only exit was blocked by the new crowds pouring into the hall. I clutched my loot and crawled out beneath the heavy, wild and blind feet. I sustained a few black and blue marks but I was still whole, alive.

Soon I was admitted to a makeshift military hospital. There I accused my friends of hiding my mother's letters. I stated that, "My mother had written to me, that my whole family was home and waiting for me. All the vases at home are full of lilacs, which wilt so fast....I have to get home with the first train." I cried, complained and an ambulance was called. The Army doctor found that my temperature was 106 F and that I had typhus. I screamed and kicked the doctor. I thought he was lying just to scare me. Typhus meant death and I was not going to die, not after having survived the camps.

I was driven to the hospital by the US medics. I was turned away by the nun/ nurse because they had no beds for females. I was puzzled and tried desperately to make sense of this statement. I had forgotten that there were two different sexes. The nurse would have been as incomprehensible to me if she had denied me admission because the walls were blue. The nun did take pity on me and offered to bathe me before I was transported to a hospital for women.

Two nuns put me in a tub of soothing warm water, holding me and washing me like a baby. They commiserated over my emaciated body covered with wounds, "Oh, you poor child! Am I hurting you with the sponge? Skin and bones, skin and bones." I started to feel sorry for myself and began to cry. Somebody was showing compassion and pity for me. This was a long forgotten experience. The guards had been threatening and cruel, outsiders indifferent and my fellow prisoners too absorbed in their own pain to spare any feeling for others.

Anna, who also suffered from typhus, joined me in the hospital. We were both near death. Miraculously we both survived. We received the best care the US Army had to offer. We were released to a camp for displaced persons and waited for organized transport home. There were negotiations going on as to how to transport the liberated masses from the US to the Soviet zone. We waited three months for a resolution of this matter.

The Russians marched into our camp. We welcomed them as our new liberators. The next day the commander politely asked us if we could walk 12 km to the train to Budapest. Most of us agreed with great enthusiasm. In one hour we were on our way to the East. There were no trains, not that day or the next. We had no food or shelter but we kept on walking. We were comforted by the direction of our march, each step brought us closer to home. There was, however, a disturbing occurrence. The Russian soldiers shot at us when we tried to grab some potatoes from the Austrian farmers' fields. We were treated again as prisoners.

After 12 days of marching we reached St. Polten where our direction was suddenly reversed. The order was 50 km to the West to the train. Some people refused to turn, started to move eastward and were shot by the soldiers. While marching next to a tall, dense cornfield, Anna and I with two friends ran into the cornfield. Fortunately we were not noticed. As the marchers passed we went to St. Polten by train through Vienna and arrived in Budapest on August 18, 1945. (Several years later I found out that our Soviet-directed march led to a train with locked cars that traveled to Siberia. A few survivors returned in 1947. Most just disappeared.)

Upon our arrival, Anna and I discovered that my brother had survived as had her son. My brother was referred to as "the poor child with no parents". I chose not to hear this comment and selected to hear, "no parents at home." I didn't ask any questions about my parents. When I had met my brother, we clung to each other and couldn't stop crying. He told me about his clever survival in a city raided by bombs, tanks and Arrowcross thugs, his daring escapes when caught with fake documents, He survived alone without money and without relatives or friends.

When Budapest was free of the Germans and the war was over, my brother went to Nagyszollos to inquire about our parents. He was not allowed in our family home by the new occupants. He wasn't allowed a souvenir, a photograph or a letter. He took a fistful of dirt from our mother's garden and brought it back in a handkerchief. Our town now belonged to the Soviet Union.

We still discussed our parents as if we were expecting their arrival. We even went to the train station to look for them among the returning deportees. Several weeks after my return, someone told me that my parents had been killed at Auschwitz. I could no longer deny their deaths. I wanted to cry but the tears wouldn't come. The self-deception had been taken away and I was empty. I couldn't cry because I had sensed for a long, long time that my parents were dead. In post-war Budapest I was unable to mourn because all of us had lost our families. The enormity of the tragedy was too great to be individually confronted so instead there was collective denial. We feverishly attempted to rebuild a new world and new lives.

My life after the Holocaust has turned out well beyond my expectations. I became an M.D. I have been happily married for 48 years. I have two children, four grandchildren, a crowd of extended family. My children are the main source of my pride and happiness. My brother and I are closer than ever.

I have habits that originated in the Holocaust. I have trouble throwing out food. I don't take simple pleasures for granted, I savor them. Whenever I take a shower I am delighted that it's warm water, not the October rain, that is running down my body. Whenever I am out in the street on a cold, rainy, windy day, I am elated, elated because soon I will be in a dry, warm, safe place. My home located on the bluest, warmest sea is that safe place.

To this day, whenever something bad happens to me I find myself counting my breaths.

With each breath I take, hope spreads inside me. As long as I can breathe, I have all the chances in the world.

Have I learned the secret that I was after? Maybe, a little part of it. I learned self-discipline, patience, compassion and humility.

May 24, 1999

Dear Judita:

It was a joy to meet with you and your husband.

I treasure the card that you gave me that depicts the barracks, the remaining chimneys of the camp, as well as the destroyed Birkenau gas chamber and crematorium chamber. I have made copies of the photographs of the Auschwitz Crematorium No. 1, of a crematorium that was perceived as inadequate because its capacity was only 700 bodies a day and of Auschwitz No. 2 (Birkenau) that was created to deal "more efficiently" with 3,000 bodies a day plus Auschwitz' prisoner overflow.

I note all the barrack chimneys that are standing alone in the Birkenau photograph. My impression is that the German population destroyed all the German-based concentration camps in 1946. Daniel Goldhagen in Hitler's Willing Executioners stated that there were not just 60, 100 or even 200 camps but rather over 10,000. He did not even want to speculate as to how many in excess of 10,000 camps existed.

I still regret that we did not get there 4 - 10 weeks earlier. It would have saved so many. I hope you realize that there were thousands of Americans, as well as other Allied forces, who were willing to fight, to sustain wounds and to die in order to destroy the horror that Hitler envisioned and realized within Europe.

With affection, gratitude and love to both of you,

George

AUSCHWITZ

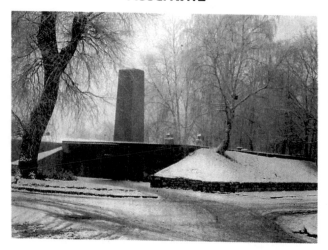

Auschwitz was the site of the first gas chamber, which was used in conjunction with cremation ovens, to facilitate mass murder. Eventually Auschwitz' gas chamber was superseded by that of Birkenau (also called "Auschwitz II") which could effect more expeditious and numerically superior numbers of deaths.

BIRKENAU

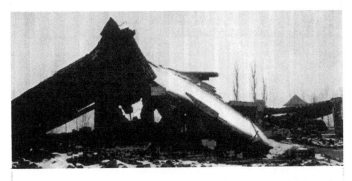

Birkenau (Auschwitz II) was largely demolished in 1945 as the Germans fled before the Russian military onslaught. A gas chamber, enclosed within a device of mass genocide, was reduced to ruins. Only remnants of this building survive as a horrific manifestation of the "Final Solution".

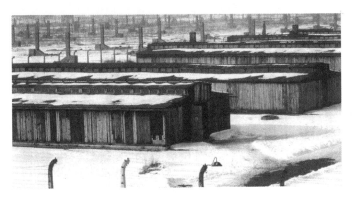

A portion of Birkenau did survive the German abandonment of the camp. In the forefront, preserved wooden barracks can be seen where the prisoners were housed. In the background are numerous chimneys, which mark the sites of dismantled or destroyed barracks.

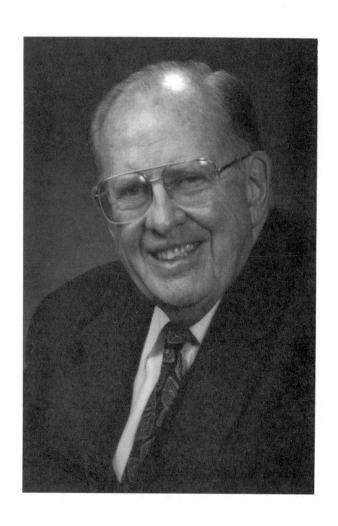

George Nicklin, M.D.

SURVIVING MASSIVE INJURIES

George Nicklin, M.D.

The hallmark of the twentieth century is immense and potential violence. I want to share how violence affected my own life and how I managed to survive. The ability to survive in the face of adversity is of practical use to all people in all societies. Adversity can be turned into a positive force. It can be used to aid not only ourselves but our fellow human beings.

People are instrumental in our attaining an ability to cope. Our parents, grandparents, great grandparents, relatives, friends and neighbors are all critical to our development. Ideally the influence of others is coupled with an innate inclination to not only survive but profit from adversity. The realization of the latter determines how successful we are in all aspects of our lives.

The ancient Chinese symbol for danger is a combination of crisis and opportunity. I have lived the Chinese curse: "May you live in interesting times." The fruition of that curse produces a very adventurous life. Life has demanded that I be incredibly courageous - at times to the point of madness. Yet God smiled on me as I passed through very dangerous terrain.

This is an account of how I survived severe injuries during World War II as an infantryman and a medical aide with the United States First Army in the Battles of France, the Bulge and Germany during the fall and winter of 1944-45. When I went into the combat zone, I had no idea that the injuries I would sustain would result in a year's hospitalization for surgical repair. I never envisioned that I would not receive psychiatric treatment for post-traumatic stress disorder. Nevertheless, I was able to benefit from this difficult experience and to use it to attain a better way of life.

I incorporated the surviving and overcoming of my injuries into my work as a psychiatrist and a mental health therapist. The following are some of the most valuable things I learned:

- Techniques for surviving a severe physical traumatic experience, such as the use of prayer.

- An awareness that psychiatric, emotional and physical effects endure for a long time after the actual injury - as long as 55 years for me.

- The effect on one's attitude to oneself - in my case as patient, physician, psychiatrist, psychoanalyst, father, human being - and to other people.

- How my desire to survive and live was affected and how my personal theology was enhanced.

- And finally how my emotional heart was enlarged

by the experience. I have a firm belief in a beneficial life plan for every human being, not restricted to today but forever.

I was born in July 1925 into an upper middle class family living in a prosperous section of the Appalachian Mountains in western Pennsylvania. My grandfather, father and paternal uncle were all engaged in the oil refining business. My mother was the sixth and youngest child of an upper middle class farmer and grain miller. My family were Anglo-Saxon Protestants in origin. I am the fourth generation on my father's side to be born in the United States and the tenth generation on my mother's side. Family members were combatants and fatalities in the American Revolution and the Civil War.

The first five years of life were eventful in several respects:

When I was around 23 months old, my sister was born. She died three months after her birth from infantile diarrhea.

At the age of 3 1/2, I contracted encephalitis believed to be Von Economo's disease or Encephalitis Lethargica or polio. I was in a coma for two weeks. The physicians believed that I would be severely brain damaged. I was not mentally damaged, but to this day the right side of my face is partially paralyzed and only my left vocal chord works.

At age five, I became aware that my father had a serious alcohol problem which caused endless irrational violent behavior against my mother and myself.

I broke my wrists three times at ages five, six and fifteen. This was important as it enabled me to understand trauma and how to weather it with an increased sense of indifference. I was accustomed to injuries by the time I entered the Army at age eighteen.

At the age of nine I discovered orgasm by accident. When I discovered that I could reduplicate it, that definitely promoted an optimistic outlook for the future. I concluded that any life system which could create such a valuable experience for humans had to have some ongoing purpose and value.

My first interest in medicine occurred at age thirteen when I was having an appendectomy. I found the hospital an interesting and stimulating place. Having just crossed the threshold of puberty, I suspect the student nurses' beauty and youth were also an impetus to my interest in medicine. Years later, during my own psychoanalysis, I became aware that if at age thirteen I perceived a hospital as an attractive place to work, this reflected on the quality of my home life.

The unexpected death of my mother when I was age fifteen (1940) strengthened my desire to become a physician. My objective was to help others avoid the agonies that I went though at that time. All my efforts were focused towards medicine as a career after this episode. My medical goal was disrupted three years later, in 1943, by World War II. I was drafted. At this time knowing I would have to fight in the war, I renounced organized religion. I felt I was not a Christian nor a Jew. I was not à Catholic nor a Protestant. I was basically an agnostic.

Upon Army induction in September 1943, I was tested and offered Infantry Officers' Candidate School. Upon inquiry I discovered that this was due to the high mortality rate of infantry officers. I opted for the college engineer training program, which would take 9 months longer plus a 3 month initial period of infantry training for the active reserve. The 9 month engineering program was canceled just as we were finishing the 3 month training for active infantry reserve. My infantry training experience started at Fort Benning, Georgia and continued in three other camps: Camp Livingston, Louisiana; Fort Mead, Maryland and Camp Kilmer, New Jersey. From New Jersey, I went across the ocean on the Queen Elizabeth I.

In late September 1944 I found myself, with 17,499 other United States soldiers, aboard the large Cunard liner Queen Elizabeth I, then the largest ship in the world. The ship had sailed with as many as 30,000 troops on board in past crossings from the United States to Northern Ireland and England. In the early years of the war it was double and triple loaded. On this ship one or two decks were double loaded, that is two men to a bunk. Triple loaded meant three men to a bunk, so that each took turns sleeping in 8 hour shifts. We ate in two shifts per day. During the crossing we spent many hours daily waiting in chow lines. All the meals were the same - crackers and creamed beef, coffee, tea or milk and maybe some vegetables or potatoes.

As the ship pulled out and arrived at the 3 mark in New York Harbor, a small vessel pulled up to the side of the ship and a distinguished passenger boarded. He was taking the Queen Elizabeth I back to England as it was the safest way to travel and was believed to be submarine-proof. It was Winston Churchill, who had just finished conferencing with Franklin D. Roosevelt.

The ship was divided into three areas - red, white and blue. Soldiers were to stay in the bow, midships or stern, depending on the color assigned to them on a tag which all troops were required to wear. I was in the white area - midships. I discovered that you could wander freely into the red and blue areas. I explored the ship. The ship was believed to be torpedo-proof because of its great speed and zig-zag course. No submarine could sink her - and I believed it. I never thought of the incredible risk the Americans and British were taking if they should be wrong.

There would have been 20,000 fatalities (including the crew) if the ship was sunk. Winston Churchill and the officers were on the upper decks, enlisted men on lower decks. Eight other "dog faces" (infantrymen) were with me in a tiny nine-bunk cabin without portholes. We were five or six levels below the water line. I got to know two of these men quite well - one from Maine (Smith - not his real name) and one from Massachusetts (Jones - also not his real name).

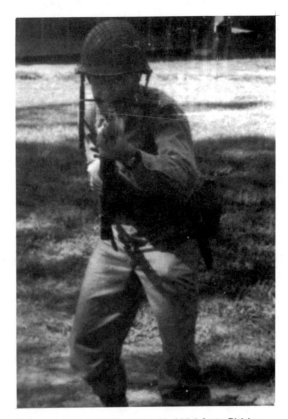

Photo courtesy of: Pvt. David Herold, 86th Infantry Division

Pvt. George Nicklin
September 1944

...with bayonet and rifle, trench knife in mouth, steel helmet, ready for replacement via Omaha Beach to front lines in Germany with 9th Division, 47th Regiment, "K" Company after six months with 86th Infantry Division at Camp Livingston, Alexandria, Louisiana hoping to meet Hitler!

I would say that they were the first psychiatric patients I ever saw in the role of a psychiatrist. Smith and Jones were both in their mid-thirties. Smith confided in me that he felt intense guilt over marrying the mill owner's daughter. Smith was especially upset that he was promoted via marriage to deputy manager of the mill. He was overwhelmed by the responsibility and heavily stressed. The Army was a break, but he would have to go back (If he survived - all of us tended to deny the possibility of our death).

Jones revealed a very important insight. He worked in a Massachusetts textile mill. He supervised several hundred women who ran the textile machinery. He was married and had one or two children with his wife. He found himself drawn to one of his supervisees and had an affair with her lasting many months. Eventually it ended. One day a colleague who knew of the affair mentioned it to him. He said to him, "Your wife certainly was wonderful about it." Jones said, "What do you mean?" The colleague replied, "She was patiently waiting for you to return. She knew you would."

Jones was dumbfounded. He could not believe it. He went to his wife and gingerly inquired if she knew. She said, "Well, I know the day that it began." She then cited the exact day. He said, "How did you know?" She replied, "I knew from the way ;you behaved that night when you came home from a 'special mill conference'. It was some months before I knew her name, but eventually I did. Throughout this I knew you would work it through and come back to me." Jones was amazed. He could not believe his wife knew the day it began and ended. He hugged his wife and thanked her from the bottom of his heart and thanked God for the episode's resolution.

I listened to these two New Englanders describe their basically very human dilemmas, which they had left behind as they went off to war. I do not know if they survived or not, but it was one of the wonders of the crossing.

One day I wandered into the chaplain's section of the ship. No one was there. There were three wicker baskets on the table filled with religious objects. One was full of crosses - Protestant! I had been raised as a Protestant and left at 17 because of pronounced hypocrisy. Next was Catholic - crucifixes! That too, I knew from my upbringing by a Catholic nanny, was subject to hypocrisy. The third basket was full of plastic tubes onto which the letter "H" was inscribed. It said on a little note in front of the basket, "Mezuza." (It contained a scroll on which the words of Deuteronomy Chapter 6, verses 4-9 and Chapter 11, verses 13-21 were written in Hebrew: "Hear, O Israel: The Lord our God is one Lord: ... And thou shall write them upon the posts of the house, and upon thy gates. ... ").

I was skeptical of the first two, but knew little of the last one. It said the "H" was the Hebrew letter shin or God. The tube had a plastic link on it so it could be put on my dog-tag chain. That was on or about September 27, 1944. It remained on my dog-tag chain until February 18, 1945, when I noticed it was missing. The plastic link that had held it to my dog-tag chain had worn through. The memory of the Mezuza and its message, however, stayed with me.

After boarding I landed in Greenoch, Scotland by lighter, (which was a small boat) and then traveled by train to a replacement depot at Nantwich, England. I crossed the Channel on the S.S. Leopoldville with about 5,000 other troops, and landed October 12th at Omaha Beach. The S.S. Leopoldville was sunk, five trips later; the crew and about 800 soldiers were lost. From Omaha Beach we traveled by rail to LeMans, France, then by truck to Liege, Belgium. The last leg of our journey left us at the front near Schevenhuette (Huertgen Forest), Germany which is on the Roer River. On October 22nd I was assigned to the Ninth Infantry Division, 47th Regiment, King ("K") Company, which at the time was the most advanced Allied unit in Germany.

There then ensued four months of intense infantry fighting - from October 22, 1944 until February 19, 1945. During this time the 120 man unit, "K" Company, was replaced with about 500 additional soldiers. The only way in which one could leave combat was to be wounded, crazy or dead. There was no rotation during that time. I was amazed to find a few men who had survived and who had been returned from the hospital. They had been part of the original landing party in Morocco, Africa in 1942 .

After my initial arrival on the Front, there was a brief period of intense fighting and then a lull. The lull was to enable Allied troops to complete the absorption of a large pocket of German troops in Aachen. On November 15, 1944 the push to Cologne resumed and my unit continued with the intention of taking several villages and towns along the rail line to the east of Aachen. It was my first major attack. We were in a forest on the northeast side of the village of Hamich. During the first four hours in the forest, my unit of 120 was cut to 65 men. The number of wounded, dead and crazy seemed incredible. I was very scared. The bombardments seemed endless. Under great stress, I found myself praying. I could not stop shaking for three days. From the number of dead appearing around me, I quickly found myself at stage three of Elizabeth Kuebler Ross' *Psychologic Stages that Precede Dying* . I proceeded to a new sixth stage, which was psychologically crucial.

Ross' five stages are:

1. Couldn't be me.
2. Rage at God, Faith, Nature, whatever made this occur.
3. Bargaining with God, Faith, Nature for reprieve,
4. Cognitive depression at seeing the reality of it.
5. Acceptance.

and my Sixth Stage is:

6. Awareness of the divine purpose of living and dying leading to peace of mind. In laying down one's life in war or peace, one contributes to God's Divine Plan, especially if perceived on God's "right" side.

During this period I experienced a sense that something divine had occurred inside of me and that I could rest assured that I would survive, with much to do upon my return home. Concurrently I was shaking uncontrollably and continued to do so for another 72 hours. I could not sleep for this 72 hour period. We feared German counterattacks during the night. Shaking was from fear and anxiety, which although better, was still unresolved. Subsequently, a calmness came over me which is called by the military, "Combat Hardened" from passing through this psychologic stress response. Such a hardened soldier can face death with equanimity. My attitude was "I will survive!" I was willing to lay down my life to open the path to the future for society. The military loves these "Hardened Soldiers".

This was my first massive psychiatric exposure. It did not move me toward the field, but it did make me aware. When I found myself in the midst of very heavy military battle in Germany, I noted, as our 120-man unit sustained repeated casualties and replacements, that about 1/3 of the casualties were psychiatric. It seemed bizarre to me when I later realized that those who stayed and fought in this madness called war were regarded as sane and those who broke down psychologically were regarded as insane. Their breakdown led to survival, which seemed sane. Sanity, defined as "staying in combat", led to death or injury for those who remained, which seemed insane. Within this *Catch 22* environment there were only four exits provided: Death, Injury, Madness or Survival To the War's End - the fourth exit being virtually impossible as we had 125 casualties per month for a 120- man unit.

The following is a quotation from General Omar Bradley, who was General Eisenhower's assistant. He was regarded as very in-tune to the problem of being an infantryman: "The rifleman trudges into battle knowing that the statistics are staked against his survival. He fights without either promise of reward or relief; behind every river is another hill - and behind that hill, another river. After weeks and months on the line, only a wound can offer him the comfort of safety, shelter and a bed. Those who are left to fight, fight on to evade death by knowing that with each day of evasion, they have exhausted one more chance for survival. Sooner or later, unless victory comes, the chase must end on the litter or in the grave."

November fighting continued with the unit being cut to 35 men. I was rotated back for a week from the front line. During that week our unit received an additional 100 men as replacements. On December 16th, I was ordered to transfer to the Medical Corps (which I had strongly resisted as medics have the highest casualty rate in combat) since I had one term of university premedical training before I was drafted. The Battle of the Bulge had begun so all my early patients were German paratroopers from the German Bulge paratroop drop. After a week of training with the captured German paratroopers and U.S. soldiers as patients, I was rotated back into the same Company and continued with them fighting the Battle of the Bulge and later the second Battle of the Rhineland, which began in late January 1945. During the four months of heavy fighting and rough winter that I was with "K' Company, the Company had about 500 replacements. I was to be the 500th member of the unit replaced.

On February 18th, 1945 my unit was moved in to replace the 82nd Airborne Division on the east side of the town of Schmidt, adjoining the Roer River and the infamous Huertgen Forest. On the morning of the 19th of February 1945, in a highly exposed position the officers ordered hot food sent to the men on the front lines. I pro-

tested to my lieutenant that this would produce casualties. I had also, during the preceding night while awaiting
the morning, had a dream - which was the last of many
dreams about fighting while in combat. It was the only
dream in which I had been shot. I awoke in the dream
having been shot. Retrospectively, I felt that this was a
clairvoyant dream that subliminally sensed the danger of
the situation.

About 8:00 AM, hot breakfast canisters were brought
up and a chow line formed in the Huertgen Forest. The
Germans could look directly at our position from the high
hill immediately on the east side of the river. I refused to
leave my foxhole for food and was enjoying my "C" ra-
tions while mortar shells could be heard fired and dropped
in our area. Immediately there was a call for "Medic". I
went out to render medical aid and had a strong sense
that shells were coming directly at me. I hit the ground.

There were a large number of shell bursts all around
me including in the trees overhead. After a minute when
the firing ended, I was unaware of any injury to myself
and proceeded to get up to go on. But in getting up, I
noticed that my left wrist was broken and clearly shrapnel
had entered the wrist joint. I crawled into a dugout with
two other soldiers, one of whom began cutting my clothes
off. I appeared to have a large number of wounds further
up my left arm and as the clothing was removed, on my
back and lower back area, lower buttocks and left leg. It
was apparent that I had received many shrapnel wounds.
Initially there was no pain. Pain arrived later. I was evacuated by stretcher. Oddly enough the man whom I had

been called to see had a minor leg wound and was one of those who had to assist in carrying me back. The barrage had eliminated about one quarter (1/4) of the unit's well-trained men who had lined up for breakfast that morning.

Real Castration Anxiety

I was taken by jeep to a collecting station and was given a pint of plasma. I never did receive a blood transfusion during my period of injury or recovery. Luckily my many wounds did not bleed profusely. I was taken eventually to the 102nd Evacuation Hospital in Aachen. It required 12 hours to arrive there. I found myself in a tent with what seemed like multitudes of wounded. I was extremely worried about surviving the 12 hour trip to the hospital. I knew from my experience as a medic that of those people who die from their wounds, 99% of them die before reaching a hospital. I seemed to have many wounds.

A young physician came and examined me. After looking me over he said that I had multiple wounds including seven wounds of my testes. I had been hit with seven pieces of shrapnel in the testicles. When I learned this, I pleaded with the young physician, "Please don't cut my balls off! I want to go back to the States and make babies." I was aware of the gangrene risk. He said, "We'll do our best."

Eventually I was taken to the operating room, given a general anesthetic and was on the operating table for about five hours while the surgical team removed 25 pieces of accessible larger shrapnel and by x-ray left thirty pieces in me. I had been wounded 55 times with shrapnel. This I learned when the surgeon came to see me the following morning. Despite being badly hurt, my attitude was very optimistic. I believe this attitude was crucial to my recovery. I prayed continuously in combat - and continued to do so. I believed this helped. God did not forsake me.

Consequences

I did not realize how serious my injuries were. It happened so rapidly that it bypassed the "pain gate." I was immobile because I had shrapnel in my left leg, left side and the middle of my back - from my left knee up to my neck.

Most of the wounds were on the left side of my body - my left arm from the upper arm to the wrist had multiple wounds, my left lung, intestines (without apparent perforation), left kidney, left buttocks, both testicles and my left thigh. A piece of shrapnel in the left lung was about three cm. below the apex of the heart. The only bones fractured and the only nerves severed were in the left wrist. I also sustained injuries in the mid-line which was directly over the spine. I now believe that the Mezuza protected me though my injuries were extremely serious.

I was so heavily bandaged that I could not effectively feed myself, go to the bathroom or do anything. My entire left arm and left leg were immobilized and I was bandaged from slightly above the left knee to just below my shoulders on the back side of the body. I was not able to walk for about six weeks after the injuries. During the first week, I was transferred from the 102nd Evacuation Hospital to a hospital train, which took me to Paris. Then I was in the Fifth General Hospital for two days - and there I had my first bowel movement which was seven days after the injuries. I was then moved to Orly Airport where I spent two days on my stretcher on the waiting room floor, along with many other American wounded. Then, after being loaded by German prisoners of war, I was flown in a DC3 to Shrewsbury, England and moved to the U.S. 155th General Hospital at Greater Malverne. I remained for three months and had two further surgical procedures. These were to debride my wounds and to recast me. The cast was removed from my left arm. There was a hole the size of half a grapefruit above my left elbow on the back of my arm. It has healed well - with a large scar. In my new awareness, I was speechless.

While in the 155th General Hospital in England I encountered two other veterans multiply wounded. One had received about 250 pieces of shrapnel. The other about 200 pieces of shrapnel. Both had absorbed heavy assault by anti-personnel mines. Neither mentioned genital injuries. I would now presume that both had them. Men do not readily speak of this.

I had one other remaining open wound on the left leg that remained open until late June 1945 after my return to the United States. I was sent back to the United States on the Moore-MacCormick ship, S.S. Brazil, with about three thousand other wounded - the leftovers of combat. Looking back my medical care was excellent. Newly discovered penicillin saved me.

I began a new life adventure as the hospital ship docked at Staten Island - a year in the hospitals of the United States Army! I was taken to Halloran Army Hospital (now Staten Island Community College) and remained there for nine months. The Mezuza continued to protect me.

It took a series of operations to get me back into good order. During the period spent at Halloran I had two more operations on my left wrist to attempt to repair the median nerve. Amazingly, today I show no signs of serious injury. More importantly my recovery allowed me to work in the orthopedic cast room for occupational therapy as a medic for rehabilitation purposes. This was made possible by an orthopedic surgeon, John Sharp, M.D., who was my cousin! I had a good experience in the hospital and greatly enjoyed getting to know the medical personnel and working in the cast room and laboratory, which was about 20% German medics, prisoners of war.

I was able to return to college in September of 1945 on convalescent furlough. This concept of letting a patient go out and do convalescent activity in the community, instead of the hospital, was a most unorthodox arrangement at that time. It took a lot of pressure, primarily from me, to convince the physicians that this was a good idea. I came to the hospital at Thanksgiving and Christmas for checkups and final operations. I was discharged from the hospital and the Army on February 5th, 1946.

The positive experiences that occurred in the hospital and while on convalescent furlough were enhanced by receipt of a letter from President Harry Truman. It seemed bizarre at that time. I was just a "dog-face."

President Truman expressed his gratitude for my valor-
ous efforts during my 121 days in combat on the front.
He hoped I would continue these efforts as a civilian to
help rehabilitate the country.

It was noted in the biography of Harry Truman, whose
World War I artillery unit sustained zero casualties, that he
had immense respect for the infantry. He realized that
military victory was dependent upon the infantry's secur-
ing and holding enemy territory. In contrast, the artillery
was always one to five miles behind the front. It was
pointed out that very few men in an offensive win the
battle. This is because one man is point and the other
men in the squad (six to twelve of them) follow directly
behind the one soldier in a dispersed line. In a front line of
thirty miles, there may be between 100 and 300 men who
are point. The whole offensive is dependent upon the
point man being there and being able to hold on in an
advance. If the spearheading infantry many are wounded
or killed, their replacement is crucial for offensive effective-
ness. It is a very small group of lowest ranked soldiers
with hundreds of soldiers coming behind them who win a
war. It is this small crucial group who actually make the
winning possible. They have high casualty and replacement rates.

In January 1946 I suffered from profound depression.
I realized I was going to be discharged from the Armed
Services and would lose its sheltering aspect. This had been
a great source of reassurance during the past two and
one half years, with the bed, board, clothing, medical care,
stipend and a blood brotherhood of fellow wounded.

Letter from President Harry Truman

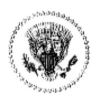

GEORGE L. NICKLIN JR., PFC. 33 801 232

To you who answered the call of your country and served in its Armed Forces to bring about the total defeat of the enemy, I extend the heartfelt thanks of a grateful Nation. As one of the Nation's finest, you undertook the most severe task one can be called upon to perform. Because you demonstrated the fortitude, resourcefulness and calm judgment necessary to carry out that task, we now look to you for leadership and example in further exalting our country in peace.

Harry Truman

THE WHITE HOUSE

164

Upon my return to the academic environment I continued to have an interest in religion and was examining different types of religion. In the fall of 1946 I discovered the Quakers. They observed a religion compatible with my personal beliefs. They had no fixed creed, no clergy, no fund solicitation and were practicing mystics. Additionally, they had no set religious format other than meditation. This seemed to parallel my beliefs which had changed that morning in November of 1944 as I confronted death. This non-creedal stance attracted a wide variety of religious views ranging from non-Christian to Christian. Their image was that of another Christian Protestant sect. This was not strictly true. Their circle of theologic love was big enough to include both non-Christian and Christians. Their God was beyond sectarian.

Psychiatry

In medical school I had become interested in psychiatry. However, going through a rotation at the New York State Psychiatric Institute, I was so appalled at the psychiatric physical machinations of that time (1950) that I could not engage in psychiatry as a specialty. I went into a family medicine residency. I was interested in surgery but felt with my injuries I could not do surgery. One third of the way through the family medicine rotation I realized that two thirds of all general medicine is psychiatry. I decided to go back to specialize in it. I consequently went to Bellevue Hospital. At that time Bellevue's psychiatric division was annually admitting 18-20,000 patients. This made it one of the busiest psychiatric "museums" in the country.

I went to the William A. White Psychoanalytic Institute in New York for my psychoanalytic training. I was attracted to it by its interpersonal orientation. I had also decided to have some psychoanalysis when I was in medical school and had a year of orthodox Freudian analysis with a member of the New York Psychoanalytic Institute. I was impressed by the proximity of the analyst technique to stimulus deprivation in this four and five hours a week analysis. This stimulus deprivation was common in "orthodox" psychoanalysis during that era. It effectively moved me in the direction of interpersonal psychoanalysis which was a more active and more effective therapeutic relationship to me.

Coping with More Castration Anxiety

I had actual castration anxiety on my mind. My seven times wounded testes seemed all right. But would they work when needed? I continued with my medical courses, marrying in 1950 and finishing medical school in 1951.

I did not realize until I was in what is now called First Year Residency, trying to do a family medicine program, that my wife and I had any problem with reproduction.   My testicles had been saved. After we had been married about a year, we tried to have children. No children appeared. Since we were aware of my injuries I went for tests. The tests indicated a sperm count of 1.25 million. Mathematically I was sterile. You need at least 40 million sperm per cc for fertility. The Germans had, for all practical purposes, castrated me.

Robert Hotchkiss, M.D. of New York University School of Medicine, one of the most experienced people in male infertility, conducted additional tests. Dr. Hotchkiss advised us to be more scientific about our reproductive efforts. He told us to have intercourse only twice a week (we had been having it usually twice a day) to conserve sperm. He said, "If you follow this in ninety days you will be pregnant." In ninety days we were pregnant. As to our current baby situation (recalling that I had stated to that U.S. physician in the 102nd Evacuation Hospital that I wanted to "go back to the States and make babies") - we have four children and eleven grandchildren - at this time.

GEORGE & KATE NICKLIN'S 11 GRANDCHIL-

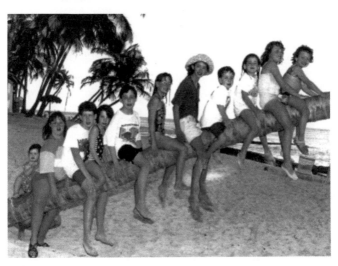

Family reunion - Club Med, Dominican Republic 1996

Neurotic Phenomena

In my experience with my personal analysis we did not talk about my real castration anxiety. We talked about the impact of my family, especially my mother, on the first fifteen years of my life. To replace my dead sister, my mother dressed me as a girl for a few months at the age of two.

During my five year training analysis I had two dreams, both based on my combat experiences.

Dream A: I was standing and juggling six round objects in the air. It turns out that these were male heads. I was very uneasy about keeping them all properly in the air.

Association A: When I was in combat one of the soldiers I was with became psychotic. This was precipitated by an acute stress reaction when his foxhole buddy had his head blown off by a shell. The head plunked into my friend's lap. While this created the roots of the dream, the actual juggling was tied up with the multiple male personalities that I had to carry in my various roles as father, husband, physician, analyst, teacher, etc.

Dream B: The second dream occurred towards the end of my analysis. In it I was flying a small Piper Cub plane. The plane had been badly shot up with many holes in the wings, fuselage and tail. I barely managed to land it on a small strip of land just behind the front lines.

Association B: This was about psychoanalytic training. The plane was my own psychoanalytic experience in training. It had so many holes in it because of the various tensions that I had discovered in myself and also those in the psychoanalytic movement. I felt that I had barely survived the various shots that had been taken at my flying machine as I was passing through the analytic training experience and existing within the various analytic groups.

Post-traumatic Stress Disorder

I do have some residual post traumatic stress disorder. If a car back-fires I have a strong desire to dive under a table or a bed. I also have some continuous daily pain as a result of my injuries. My attitude is stoic. Deny the pain! Try to maintain a high threshold of resistance to pain. Be optimistic!

One of these post-traumatic stress symptoms was manifest in a dream I had in the last eight years.

Dream C: I was fighting hand-to-hand with a German. He had his arm around my neck from behind me. I managed to get his arm into my mouth and took a good, stiff bite out of his forearm. He began yelling loudly.

It was the middle of the night and my wife and I were both asleep in bed. My wife had her arm underneath my head. She had gotten her forearm by my mouth. I woke up and found my wife yelling loudly. I had just bitten her in the arm.

This kind of dream does occur, although I have not had one now for a few years. My residual post-traumatic stress disorder episodes have become less and less frequent as the years have gone on. When a car backfires I still feel that I should duck. When I look out over a vista of trees I sometimes wonder if someone lurks behind with a gun. I am sure this is residual from my fighting experiences in World War II.

What Enhanced My Recovery?

- I prayed silently many times daily.
- I had a mystical experience about November 25th, 1944. God said, "You will survive!" - I had great <u>hope</u>.
- I felt what I was doing was crucial for the world's future - especially for the United Nations' founding and for Jewish survival.
- Hitler retreated every one of the 121 days I was there!

Attitude

An interesting phenomenon that has come out of the war is my optimism. I believe this is related to my surviving the 55 pieces of shrapnel that hit me. If I could successfully contend with massive injuries; I could contend with almost anything. I also feel that the world is basically good, my life is good, the future is good and God has been good to me. I'm a little "holeyer" than thou, maybe even holier than thou!

Is Self Divulgence Useful in Therapy?

It is my general impression that most therapists do not want to be self-divulgent with patients but prefer to concentrate on the patient's situation. I feel it is useful for a therapist to be empathetically self-divulgent with a patient, especially in cases that seem hopeless. For instance, a patient came in after many years of therapy with another therapist which had left her seriously damaged. Early in therapy there was a comment by the patient that, "you probably have had no awareness of such problems." I shared with the patient that I had been severely injured in

World War II which required one year's hospitalization and that there was definitely hope for her recovery. I knew recovery was possible. This patient eventually showed marked improvement and a very significant recovery from disabilities. With other patients who have questioned their ability to survive in society, I have shared my survival history. These patients later stated that it was encouraging to realize that it was possible to survive effectively .

One of the major aspects of therapy is hope. The therapist must offer realistic hope to a patient to assist in recovery. It is the search for hope that drives patients into the office. Our personality should clearly communicate that sense of hope to the patient. It is through my own recovery from disabilities that hope is communicated. My personal analysis plays a significant role in this with each patient I come in contact with. Each adversity is a potential opportunity.

What is the Gain?

The following principles evolved from my World War II experiences:

1. Medical Care Providers

I was humbled and helped by seeing the role of aides, nurses and physicians in the recovery of seriously injured patients. My war contact with aides and nurses made me aware that they are very valuable people. Studies have validated this. They have more patient contact than physicians. The physician's contact is certainly valuable but more intense and brief. The demands for medical care are both intensified and diversified by the massive influx of casualties during war. For example, Halloran Hospital's cast room treated 100+ wounded persons per day, as hospital ships docked weekly from Europe. There was an incredible demand for competent and expeditious care. All levels of the health profession had to be responsive.

2. A Special Time Concept.

We have a limited amount of time to live. It is well to consider how many hours this is - currently it is approximately 666,000 hours or 76 years. We are programmed to biologically destruct at around the 666,000th hour but may live for an extra 100,000 or more hours if we are fortunate. (There are 876,000 hours in a century.)

We can understand how short this is. How important it is that we utilize this limited amount of hours. Aware of the length of time we are here, we have a responsibility to make the best of our lives and of each hour that we are alive.

3. Future Ideal Imperative

I believe I have discovered a principle, which I call the Future Ideal Imperative. In the immediate present all human beings are basically motivated by what they perceive to be the thought or act that will bring the greatest beneficial consequence not only to themselves, but to their families and the other people beyond their family structure. This includes village, city, state, nation and world. This is now being manifested in a concern about space and the other planets, etc. Obviously the awareness is expanding and is affecting our daily, hourly and minute decision-making process. It includes such considerations as: cholesterol, smoking, alcohol, drugs, nuclear power, and space exploration, etc.

4. The Cascade of Generations

We are increasingly aware of time. This is a new perception. There is an overview of about 250 years while we are alive. You have a personal knowledge of people who have lived during this 250 year span. You may ask, "How can this be?" The answer is that we are aware of our grandparents, who in today's world can expect to live about 80 years. My grandparents were born in 1860 and their grandparents, of whom I have photographs, were born in England in 1796. We likewise will live about 80 years and we will also be aware of our children and grandchildren and possibly even our great grandchildren, who will live into about the year 2110 A.D. This overview of time, 1860 to 2110, is 250 years yet it may be as little as 220 or as many as 270 years or more.

Consideration of a generational cascade causes a better perspective of time - past, present and future. New methods of data will allow a record not only of pictures but of the pictorial subject's speech and movement. This data can be readily accessed by future generations. My grandparents, parents, myself, my wife and our children have been educated in order to achieve a better present and future. None of us have planned for just our immediate life. We have planned for those around us and our direct progeny. In the United States Presidency we plan for four years or eight years. I believe we must begin to plan for 100 years ahead, 200 years ahead, etc. Decisions that we make today, such as nuclear pollution, will affect people's lives for hundreds of thousands of years to come. This realization must accompany an awareness of our place and responsibilities within the cascade of generations.

5. Brain Life-Plan Center

I believe that in the brain of each human being is a life-plan center consisting of a few cells. It may or may not be in our consciousness. This center plans on data input - not just for today but forever. Do I know where in the brain? No I do not know where, but I believe there is such a center, a conglomerate of cells that does this long-range planning. I believe we see it at work in our scientific research and our medical research, market forces, birthrate, etc., etc.

6. Adversity Sublimation into Creating Education for the Future

All the forces, operative in me, compelled me to become active in various educational pursuits - from pre-K through graduate education.

The purpose of education is to produce graduates who can live constructively in the 21st century, in the third millennium and beyond. These future graduates will be aware, as many of us are, of their own culture and of at least two additional culture units. They will speak two other languages besides their native language allowing them to swiftly and effectively move around the world. This is long-range planning. Stop a moment to consider your own long-range planning. Assimilation of the individual occurs ideally within the parameters of the entire globe.

Do I still have feelings about the Mezuza? Yes, I do. In my office and residence, there are three Mezuzas. One guards the entrance, two are on doorways within the house. Do I think they make a difference? We all want to delay the Angel of Death. I know that Angel passed me by in Germany as centuries earlier the Jews of Egypt escaped the Angel, who spread death within the homes of the Egyptians. The Mezuza's message has been realized during my life: "That your days may be multiplied, and the days of your children, in the land which the Lord sware unto your fathers to give them, as the days of heaven upon the earth." Even my injuries were a gift from God.

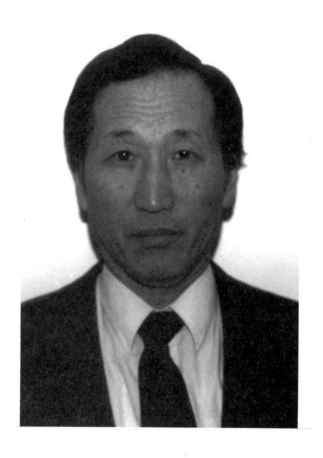

Hae Ahm Kim, M.D.

PULMONARY TUBERCULOSIS, WAR, IDEOLOGY and PSYCHOANALYSIS

Hae Ahm Kim, M.D.

"Bombs were falling all around us and my
Pearl was dying; she had high fever, delirious
and was calling your name, haeam, haeam"
"What's wrong?" "Three men in black cape
are trying to abduct me, I don't want to go
and they are forcing me, help, help".

Pearl had three days of agonizing toxic hallucinations before succumbing to death at the tender age of seventeen. Her mother carried her emaciated body with the help of two men she was able to hire, to a nearby makeshift cemetery. She was buried in a shallow grave among many war casualties. War was raging and bombs were still falling.

This is the account Pearl's mother gave me when I met her about six months after the Korean War ended. Pearl had endured for almost three years with miliary tuberculosis, a fulminating form of tuberculosis. She finally succumbed to it a few months before the war ended. Lack of proper nutrition and modern medicine allowed her illness to spread to peritonitis and become toxic. She suffered from terrible toxic hallucinations as described by her mother. Pearl was the only child her mother had and they had been caught under fire near the landing zone in the last few days of her life. The mother lamented that had the daughter lived a few months longer, she could have gotten the benefit of modern medicine which came with the arrival of the U.S. military forces in Inchon, South Korea.

Three years earlier, I had caught tuberculosis. It started with pleural effusion and loss of weight. The school physician advised me to take a leave of one year to restore my health. I was on the family farm for about four months when I heard the war sound. It was tragic that both Pearl and I were victims of tuberculosis. I, however, survived and had survivor's guilt for some time and tried to appease it by trying to retrace her whereabouts during her last few months of life. I remember I had such sorrow to be alive.

During the post-World War II era, Korea was recovering from devastation with the help of American economic aid. People, however, were still starving and nutrition was poor. The spread of tuberculosis was rampant despite new methods of chemotherapy with Streptomycin, Isoniazid and Para-aminobenzoic acid. Young men and women were afflicted with tuberculosis and the best method of treatment at the time was isolation and aggressive chemotherapy which the majority of patients were not able to afford.

During the summer of 1950 we were again starving. This was during the Korean War so soon after World War II. Our family was regarded as capitalist by the invaders, who ordered us to vacate our house in favor of our worker's family who only pretended to take it over. We were able to hide on the farm and were not sent fifty miles away. We survived on farm produce such as pears, melons, and apples with some smuggled in grains. Although my nutrition was rather poor, exercise restored my health. By the end of 1950, we had to evacuate to the south by train as the Chinese invasion of the Korean peninsula occurred.

Both Verdi in *La Traviata* and Puccini in *La Boheme* have romanticized consumption. As Romeo and Juliet did, Marguerite Gautier, the Lady of the Camellias in *La Traviata* made her love for Armand so noble and self-sacrificing that their love exceeded others. It makes the love universal and cosmic, a love which transcends and indeed is oblivious to illness and inevitable death. In Puccini's *La Boheme*, young artists transcend class, wealth and other social differences making the Bohemian culture an ideal of love, creating nineteenth century romanticism. The deaths of Marguerite and Mimi in *La Boheme* are not portrayed as horrific ends to very shortened lives but as secondary consequences to the realization of romanticized love. It is the realization of love that is emphasized, death and fatal illness are reduced to dramatic backgrounds. Audiences react with a sense of sorrow and misgivings to the end of love not to the concurrent reality of death.

Thomas Mann in the *Magic Mountain* describes what it was like to be sick with tuberculosis in those years without modern treatment with chemotherapy. What is it that makes tuberculosis so romantic with dreams of adventure? Hans Castorp in the *The Magic Mountain* during a visit to his cousin, Joachim Jiemsssen in Davos, Switzerland describes the sudden and unexpected diagnosis of his tuberculosis. Castorp becomes aware that his illness is not exclusively somatic but rather is inclusive of spiritual/ psychological immaturity. Confronted by the disease and possible death, Hans develops humor, substantiation of life and extraordinary enlightenment.

As Thomas Mann said, "Holy Grail is mystery. Humanity is mystery too." Castorp is positively influenced by his seven years in the sanatorium, yet each source of influence also possesses a counter-influence. In *The Magic Mountain* each of these influences is personified in a human being who is simultaneously a personification and a complex, well-rounded, believable character in the tradition of realistic fiction.

Krokowski is an example of the superficially one-dimensional character, who in reality conveys a multi-faceted message Krokowski, the assistant to the sanitarium director Behrens, is a psychoanalyst. In general he represents Mann's opinion of psychoanalysis and Freudian theory in the early 1920s. Mann's view is not very favorable. Krokowski can be viewed as grotesque or even as a comic character. Yet in a broader sense he is a personification of Mind, balancing Behrens who represents Body. Krokowski represents the dark, the elusive, the intuitive in the human psyche, in short the unconscious, in contrast to Behrens who represents the overt and physiological aspect of the human organism. Krokowski's most important role in the novel is to deliver a series of lectures on the subject of "Love as a force contributory to disease." These lectures simply represent Mann's interpretation, or distortion, of Freudian theory as Mann perceived it in the early Twenties. It is summed up in the statement Krokowski makes in the first lecture: Symptoms of disease are nothing but disguised signs of the power of love; all sickness is only love transformed. Naturally this theory is diametrically opposed to Behrens' view of disease as organic in origin - the idea that tuberculosis is merely caused by infectious organisms and can be cured with medical means. Behrens' view, the most obvious one, is, however, oversimplified. Even though Mann is satirical or even hostile toward Krokowski, he agrees with this somewhat sinister "prophet" that many diseases begin in the soul. Mann's recognition of this concept would provide the basis for the considerable alteration in his opinion of psychoanalysis during the following years.

Pearl and I had grown up full of the hope and joy of youth - until the war came. More than half of my 17 and 18 year old high school classmates were drafted and perished in the war. Many of them also died from illnesses like tuberculosis. I was unfit for the military because of my tuberculosis. The war benefited me in an ironic way. Due to the rest and my country living, my health got better and I and my surviving classmates were able to return in the fall of 1953 to my high school in Pusan, closed for almost three years. I was able to return to my original class from which I had taken a year's leave of absence.

Tuberculosis is a slowly progressive not readily detectable disease which resembles chronic neurosis or character disorder. I had many friends who were afflicted with tuberculosis. Those who were ill, appeared to be meditative and philosophical; some wanting to emulate and end up like Hans Castorp. My "magic mountain" was in psychoanalysis which I did not know until I got into it years later after medical school. The more I became involved the more I was enchanted with mysteries and unknown things about humanity and the human psyche. Freud thought that psychoanalysis was a new way of looking at the unconscious process of our minds and that analysis was a tool. Tuberculosis was a mystery at one time and humanity succumbed to it. We thought that through chemotherapy we had complete control over it, but as we know now, we do not. Healing humanity is the same. We may know some ways of healing, but the mystery is too profound to grasp as yet.

Let me tell you a true story. I lived in Inchon, the seaport of Seoul with a beautiful harbor that opens into the Yellow Sea. My family lived in that town from 1945 to 1949 in a beautifully manicured home with a Japanese rock garden. I joined the United States Information Service which was situated near the western mansion called "Inchon gak" which means palasso. The curator of the service from 1945 to 1948, was Mr. Ahn. He was Korean, grew up in Shanghai and had a perfect command of English. He ran the center with culturally rich programs featuring seasonal festivities, folk song instruction, sing alongs, cowboy story telling, English oratorical contests, etc. The promotion of American-style democracy was placed in direct competition with communism.

Among the young members at the USIS, there were two outstanding members, Marvin and Michael. They were sponsored to go to America by a United States military officer who was a Lieutenant Colonel. He had come from a Midwestern state and was a farmer and an engineer. He sponsored these two bright boys who spoke English so well. None of us could compete with them. They passed all the required paperwork and examinations except the physical. Mike was all right but Marvin was found to have a "wet spot", the early phase of tuberculosis and was grounded. Michael refused to go to America alone saying that they had brotherly vows to stay together. Marvin thought that his condition would improve with treatment but it did not. His condition got worse. Marvin pleaded with Mike to go alone but he declined. Then the war came. Neither of them could go to America and Marvin got worse during the war without proper nutrition and enough medicine. I went to visit him in the hospital in Seoul in the fall of 1950 before we fled to the south after the invasion of the Chinese communists into the Korean peninsula. He looked awful but his mood was great.

Marvin lived his life until his last day as if he were in an American Midwestern town. He spoke nearly perfect English and read every magazine and newspaper in English which was available in Korea at the time. Mike was working for a high level interpreter for the United States 8th Army in Seoul and paid regular visits to Marvin.

People talked about their ill-fated stories as rose buds of war-torn Seoul. Although they were not blood related brothers, they were closer than any brothers known to anyone. Mike had many opportunities to go to America after the armistice was signed in 1953 but he did not go. Marvin died in the middle of the war in the chronic disease branch hospital of Seoul National University Hospital. I went there to visit a couple of times less than a year later. During those visits I found that Marvin's mother was a distant relative of my father. His mother was in her late fifties and I never heard from her after the war. A rumor I did hear later was that she was one of the victims of mass carpet bombing air raids by B-29's which leveled Seoul into a heap of dust. I met Michael in a U.S. military uniform in a jeep on a Seoul street working as a liaison officer. After that, I had no further contact with him.

To this date, I can not understand Marvin too well. He was a big framed man with interesting facial features: a broad forehead with thick eyebrows, light green/brown eyes and a sharp-pointed high-bridged nose which is unusual for Koreans. His mother was a very sociable and foul-mouthed woman with a big frame but not fat. She reminded me of a middle-aged Italian woman. She got a divorce when Marvin was young and never remarried which was also rare in those days. She had large round eyes with a very light brown coloring which was rare for Korean women. What did I guess about those features? Some of the early Portuguese sailors who had been shipwrecked while they were heading toward Japan ended up on Cheju Island or southern Chulla province. The

Chosun government allowed them to settle there. Some of them remained and married local women. Marvin's parents and their relatives originated from those areas.

These events in my life were part of the reason I chose psychiatry as my specialty. Psychiatry in my day was not popular at all. Until the late 1960's we learned mostly descriptive psychiatry derived from the Kroepelinian German school. Dynamic psychiatry of psychodynamics and psychoanalysis were fascinating to many psychiatric leaders in Korea at the time.

What is common between a psychiatric sanctuary and a tuberculosis sanatorium is the fact that both tuberculosis and psychoanalysis take a long time to heal and both really require a "time-out" to devote your life to the treatment of your soul and your body. The sanitarium concept is not new in psychotherapy but what it requires is devotion from both patients and therapists. The fact is that it takes a long time to heal and it is costly - a long time of separation is required from the familiar environment where the trauma occurred, a prolonged preparation for readaptation or separation on return. Human life is more complicated in a real life situation than we can possibly be prepared for.

Korea used to have large scale sanctuaries called state institutions which had self sustaining community facilities such as a patient's coop, canteen, recreational set-ups, libraries, etc. For some reason these communities were not regarded as a real community. Many adult homes have been created in the middle of towns across the nation but no better results are produced. We can draw a similarity to tuberculosis treatment through high altitude exposure in Europe in the nineteenth century. The efficiency of it was questionable but it was the best option at that time. In the environment of the sanatorium, young people became idealists and often became ardent socialists or even anarchists, claiming they had nothing much to lose because they would die soon anyway, etc.

In Korea, there was political chaos after World War II and before the Korean War broke out in 1950. Many different political parties were engaged in nasty smear campaigns and political assassinations were frequent occurrences. Young people were largely divided into two groups: one which supported western style democracy and the other which advocated socialism and communism. Student demonstrations and clashes with police were an everyday event. A chronic illness like tuberculosis and a despairing mood were a good combination to inflame youthful rebellion against the social system. North Korean agitation made the situation worse and eventually armed conflict between local communist rebels and North Korean infiltrators caused civil war strife for a couple of years prior to the Korean War.

I had a personal friend, Professor S.C. Song, who spent a few years in a sanatorium in Korea before the war, recovered from tuberculosis and got better after a lobectomy. He came to the U.S. in the late 1950s and became a linguist, receiving a Ph. D. from the University of Michigan. He wrote a Korean language syntax which became a classical scientific work. Unfortunately he died a few years ago in California from a stroke and pneumonia. He was one of those intellectual rebels who were supportive of the social causes of justice and equality. His life strengthened me.

One of the key characteristics of tuberculosis is the almost universal prediction of its dire consequences - death or a survival fight which is both spiritually and financially costly. Thomas Mann wrote, "Hans Castorp overcomes his inborn attraction to death and arrives at an understanding of humanity that does not, indeed, rationally ignore death nor scorn the dark, mysterious side of life, but takes account of it, without letting it get control over his mind. What he comes to understand is that one must go through deep experience of sickness and near death to arrive at a higher sanity and health; just the same way that one must have knowledge in order to find redemption."

I have had experience and also have observed people around me who suffered and died in war and of illnesses which give me deep sympathy with humanity. I feel the need for the healing of our mind and body. These revelations propelled me into medicine and psychiatry. A great while later, I realized that our conscious mind only controls a small part of our life. Mann further wrote, "Our consciousness is feeble; only in moments of unusual clarity and vision do we really know ourselves." Probably this kind of awareness in the preconscious mind helped me to enter psychoanalysis.

Recovery, Empathy and Psychoanalysis

I knew that recovery from tuberculosis helped me to have a stronger personality and to have better control of my own fate. In order to build better self discipline I started cold water massage every morning regardless of the season or weather conditions. I also learned to meditate and concentrate in a manner similar to transcendental meditation. The war years were my recovery period and I advanced right into study in high school in exile. I did well and entered Seoul National University and its medical school. I knew I had developed a deeper empathy than I had prior to my illness with tuberculosis. I felt for the patients who had mental illnesses and who had hallucinations like Pearl. In medical school, I already made up my mind to major in psychiatry. I was particularly touched by Da Zein psychology, existential philosophy and Binswanger's phenomenology. War brought existential issues to the intellectual minds in Korea and became popular after the downfall of communism and socialism.

I was not the only one who was ill. In the country as a whole, there was a state of shock and sickness. The country, Castorp and I had parallel life experiences. Quoting Mann , "In the hermetic, feverish atmosphere of the enchanted mountain, the ordinary stuff of which he is made undergoes a heightening process that makes him capable of adventures in sensual, moral, intellectual spheres he would never have dreamed of in the flat land. His story is the story of the heightening process itself. It employs the method of the realistic novel, but actually is not one. It passes beyond realism by means of symbols, makes a vehicle for intellectual and ideal elements." The flat land is real life and not the heightened period of war and misery. Here we find chronic illnesses called mental diseases and emotional illnesses.

I have gone through many symbolisms, and the stark reality of war made a firmer commitment to the pursuit of human psychology. I found similarities between the psychoanalytic process and the recovery from pulmonary tuberculosis; both can take years of therapy or treatment and also go through recognizably different stages. Both processes transform one's personality and bring new perspectives on life.

Hans Castorp planned to visit his cousin in the mountain's high altitude for a couple of weeks, but he remained for seven years to recover from tuberculosis which he did not know he had at the time of his visit. It seems that this is what happens often with mental illnesses: sudden unexpected illnesses, hospitalizations, suicide, acting out, etc. Thomas Mann went to visit his wife in the sanitarium for three weeks but he did not stay there. He left and wrote *The Magic Mountain*.

Benefits

What did tuberculosis do for me? It made me come to the United States and study psychoanalysis. During this period, initially I had four years of personal analysis and twenty years later two years of a second analysis . What did my analyses do for me? It helped me to overcome the myths of my life and heightened my experience for the middle years of my life. My second analysis gave me what Mann calls "Transubstantiation". He used this term in connection with the mysteries of the Holy Grail. This analysis, I felt, also gave me a clearer picture of what psychoanalysis is all about and removed the myths surrounding the

process of any analysis without extraordinary enlightenment and substantiation. I experienced it as an ordinary
human experience and not as a mysterious or magical science. I felt that I had developed the virtues of persistence
and of endurance, of a slow start and long recovery, which
are the very characteristics of tuberculosis. It takes a long
time to develop personality and mastery of one's own
senses and the discovery of self.

The Future of Psychoanalysis

Let us make another comparison. The face of tuberculosis has changed with the discovery of chemotherapy. Tuberculosis has never become extinct. The recent occurrence
of multi-drug-resistant strains of tuberculosis bacilli is an
example. There has to be constant pursuit of new methods
of treatment and the discovery of new medications.

Likewise, psychoanalysis may have changed its face but
it may never become extinct. We may have to change the
format and scale (theories and techniques) to render hu-
mane and empathic cures of human misery, however much
it takes in time and effort. I have learned through my experience of illness that essential moral and intellectual aspects
of my life have changed and matured. Through such personal experience and physical transformation one may be
freer of rigid, dogmatic and judgmental attitudes in analysis. A higher level of instinctual sublimation and spiritualiza-
tion in the analytic relationship and beyond may occur if
one should overcome the handicap whatever it may be
during the recovery. It may take analysis to work it through
and it may be worth it.

Thomas Mann explains that a foreign tongue can ease embarrassment and overcome reluctance in expressing love and affection. Hans Castorp was able to express his love in French when he felt unable to say it in German. In psychoanalysis do we use certain analytic terminology to avoid embarrassment or because we can not explain things in ordinary language? Has English become a standard language for psychoanalysis? There has been no problem for me with terminology or language once I really understood myself and psychoanalysis in a developmental perspective. Moreover, you can express love and affection in any language or beyond language without embarrassment and inhibition. In my mind this is the ultimate goal for personal analysis and self analysis for ourselves and our patients. We want to be free from the shroud and strangeness of psychoanalysis and human psyche by means of love and empathy which we earn through our own life experiences including serious illnesses. In my case it was pulmonary tuberculosis.

BIBLIOGRAPHY

Crapanzano, Vincent (1980), *Tuhami-Portrait of a Moroccan*, University of Chicago Press, Chicago, IL

Mann,Thomas (1929), *The Magic Mountain*, Vintage Books Edition, 1969 Alfred A. Kropf, Inc., New York, NY

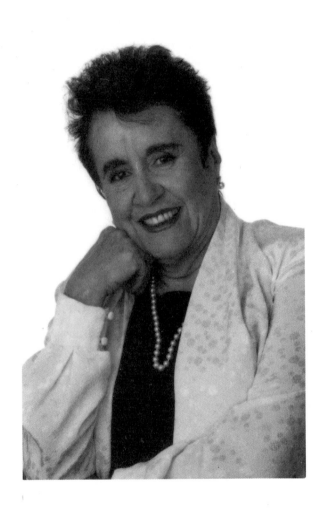

Leah Davidson, M.D.

REACTIONS TO HYSTERECTOMY REVISITED

Leah Davidson, M.D.

The French painter George Braque once re
marked, "Truth exists. Only falsehood needs
inventing." He was referring to the painter's
observing eye and to the authenticity of the painter's integrated inner vision. In a similar vein, I have recently had
cause to reexamine some of our psychoanalytic, and other
beliefs, with regard to women's reproductive organs.

I view myself as a kind of middle-aged athlete. Over
the past 25 years I have considered bodily discipline and
the preservation of stamina to be of primary importance
to both longevity and good mental health. I regard taking
good care of my body as good common sense.

A few years ago, I discovered that I was developing a
cystocoele. The cystocoele became further aggravated by
the presence of fibroids in a retroverted uterus. I therefore
went to a gynecologist, who had been recommended by
my internist. This gynecologist, although an older man,

taught in a university hospital and had a reputation for being "a women's libber". I was consequently very surprised to discover that my discomfort was not worthy of his serious consideration. His comment was: "It's only the size of an egg." His opinion was that I should tolerate both my conditions since I was now an older woman. "Conservative approaches are best," he advised. His attitude, however, towards the young, pregnant women waiting in his office was far friendlier and more energetic. In retrospect I believe that his lack of interest and his conservative advice were based more upon his inadequate surgical knowledge and fear of risk than upon my medical needs.

I sought a second opinion. Through my personal contacts, I found someone who was more in touch with my medical situation. My new gynecologist was less ageist and more sensitive to my needs. After prescribing replacement hormones, my doctor advised that surgery would certainly be beneficial. Since it was to be an elective procedure, he urged me to pick my own time and to be as emotionally prepared as possible. We discussed the clinical advantages of the vaginal hysterectomy versus abdominal approaches. My gynecologist assured me of his expertise in both vaginal hysterectomy and cystocoele repair. He demonstrated with diagrams exactly how and why he would proceed using the vaginal approach.

Throughout my exposure to this doctor, I felt respected both as a colleague and as a woman. Some of my trust in him was undeniably mixed with the positive transference I required to overcome my fear of surgery (Kernberg 1976).

194

This fear was also considerably reduced by my realistic feelings that this was indeed a competent and caring person, a person who would not unnecessarily mutilate my body or alternatively not do enough to alleviate my discomfort.

As the time for the surgery came closer, I experienced a sense of sadness and loss. This took the form of intermittent, imaginary conversations with my uterus. The dialogue followed a general pattern and included certain ideas:

Uterus:	"Why are you getting rid of me? Why do I have to die before you?"
I:	It's the bladder. You've got fibroids. You're pulling down the bladder. I am at risk for infections."
Uterus:	"I have given you children. I have served you well."
I:	"But now you grow fibroids and I am not comfortable."
Uterus:	"I am an old friend."
I:	"Even old friends have to part."
Uterus:	"Silence and sadness."

I prepared myself as best I could for the inevitable loss. I took a preoperative vacation with a friend and planned every step of the operative and post-operative recovery. I felt in charge of what was going to be a difficult, but necessary step in an ultimately constructive experience.

What I was totally unprepared for was the reaction to my impending surgery of other mental health professionals. I received 20 different reactions during the course of casual conversations with men and women. These conversations were necessitated by my need to postpone certain obligations and to make alternate arrangements.

It did not occur to me during these conversations, that I was hearing fearful, anxious or irrational responses. At the time I perceived only puzzlement and confusion. Overall what I heard from colleagues was not responsive to what I was experiencing. It was only after my operation that I felt some mild anger about having been the recipient of what I now recognize as someone else's projection. I subsequently decided to look into the phenomenon more objectively, to try to understand what had interfered with the empathic communication I come to expect from people in our field.

These are the responses of some of my colleagues to the subject of my pending hysterectomy:

Male, middle aged: "Oh! You are going to be depressed for at least a year! It's natural. Read the Jungians. You're dealing with the universal birthplace of the world."

Female, middle aged: "Why are you doing this? I don't know what I would do if I were you. I wouldn't feel like a woman." (burst into tears)

Female, middle aged: "I'll call you the minute you come out of the theater. I must know how you are."

Male, forty-five: " Well. I suppose this is the end of something important in your life. Like sexuality? Most women lose libido after a hysterectomy. It's like losing your prostrate gland. You're not the same."

Male, middle aged: "How masochistic you are! Why would you want to spend six months of your life recuperating and weak."

The above responses were qualitatively different from those of close friends or of lay people, all of whom asked more questions about the need for the operation, my preparations and other reality-based matters. These were also the people who volunteered to help and to support me. They were a marked and welcome contrast to those I now term the "psychobabblers". My surgical experience was very different from that so frighteningly portrayed by the latter group.

I went into the hospital calmly, did not require sleeping medication the night before and read a book for three hours when surgery was delayed the next morning. The procedure was painless and I returned home on the fourth post-operative day. My recovery was quick and uneventful. I did not feel depressed but there was a psychosomatic sense of "emptiness" where the uterus used to be. It was as if my body was sensing and exploring the differences and adjusting to the loss. I thought of it as a phenomenon akin to the "Phantom Limb" after amputation. I wondered if this reaction was a normal, bodily response to the loss of any organ

For approximately two weeks, I experienced a sense of accomplishment and of exhilaration at having successfully survived and realized my preoperative goals. These sensations were interspersed with a mixture of relief and gratitude for those who helped me and for existing without pain or discomfort for the first time in many years.

Concurrently I became more solicitous of the needs of my friends and more compassionate towards their difficulties in life. I wondered whether this was a reaction to losing my uterus (i.e. a substitute for mothering) or was it more simply and basically a surge of Eros over Thanatos, part of the happiness of being alive and well.

There was one other experience with regard to losing my uterus that was both significant and relevant. Prior to the surgery, I had a hypnagogic image of my uterine cervix opening. A small fairy flew out of it and took wing upwards. I understood the image to be a metaphoric communication of psyche and soma, i.e. body and soul. The uterus had borne my living children. It would now in some fashion play a part in the creative productions of my mind - that is, my "brain children". A month or so after the surgery, without any conscious preplanning, I found myself writing the outline of this piece.

Paradoxically, I also found that during the planning of my operation, the lay journalistic information which claimed to be protecting women from unnecessary surgery was often inaccurate and alarmist in its anxiety to sell copy. For example, a lengthy article overstressed the loss of some hormones after a hysterectomy, particularly testosterone. This article emphasized the resultant loss of energy which accompanies the hysterectomy ("New York" magazine, January 1988). Statistics undoubtedly prove that too many unnecessary hysterectomies are performed in the United States - 650,000 per annum. 650,000 is a conservative estimate. 530,000 hysterectomies are undertaken for non-cancerous conditions (NIH Guide, March 1996).

On the other hand, the clamor and generalizations on the protectionist end seldom help a woman make a good individual decision. The following quote from a short piece in "Modern Maturity" magazine (February - March 1989) addresses this issue: "Even more distressing are the consequences that can follow surgery: Diminished sexual enjoyment, chronic fatigue, and increased risk of heart disease and severe depression." This statement is technically correct, yet the statement is by emotional implication unbalanced. It characterizes the woman as a victim of surgical lust. It unfortunately does not inform with regard to particulars for the individual woman. The article ends with the importance of referral to a counseling clinic and a physician referral clinic. The article fails, however, to mention the invaluable first step of talking intelligently more than once to one's own physician and of planning one's own steps in the process. The article's author is currently writing a book on avoiding hysterectomy and this skew is pervasive in her writing.

A highly commendable book is *Hysterectomy: Before and After* (1988) by Winifred Cutler, Ph.D. which stresses both the need for and the dangers of hysterectomy when done unnecessarily or carelessly. Most importantly the book focuses on the detailed medical research in each relevant area and also on the importance of a good patient-doctor alliance. Likewise, several later articles also stress the need for better available information. (NIH Guide, Jan. 1995; NIH Guide, March, 1996; Toaff, Michael E.: http: / / www.netreach.net/~hysterectomyedu/ myomecto.htm, "Alternatives to Hysterectomy: Myomectomy; Toaff, Michael

E.:   http://www.netreach.net/~hysterectinyedu/ whywould.htm, "Why Would a Woman Resist Hysterectomy?")

Psychoanalytic literature, on or about women's reproductive organs, has from the very beginning suffered from a polarity between fearful awe and uninformed generalization. In contrast, the literature which has taken an accurate cognitive perspective on this issue often ignores the mythic dimension present in unconscious attitudes to the topic. The phallocentricity of Freud's theories about femininity was questioned as early as 1927 by Earnest Jones as follows: "There is a healthy suspicion growing that male analysts have been led to adopt an unduly phallocentric view of the problem in question, the importance of the female organs being correspondingly underestimated (1950)."

I do not know of many studies that explore the necessity for this phallocentric view from the anthropological perspective of fear of woman's sexual organs, particularly regarding their ability to give birth. Marvin Drellich, in a 1981 paper on female psychology, states: "In both sexes, the sexual organs may be symbolically utilized to express a variety of attitudes, positive and negative towards oneself, and other members of one's own sex. It seems to me that phallocentric theories of female development are attempts at restitution of male power when faced with the mysteries, scientific and otherwise of human conception." A common clinical phenomenon which illustrates this point is when males lose sexual interest in their partners after the birth of a child. One of my male patients, a man in his late twenties whose presenting symptom in therapy was premature ejaculation, had the following dream shortly after the birth of his first child, "I am running in the street and there is a woman running ahead of me and dropping babies out of her womb as she runs. I can't catch up with her and I feel scared."

All of us are fascinated by creation, whether depicted as an embryo on a TV screen or as the theme of an American Indian tale where man is fashioned from clay. Women experience giving birth to and raising a child as an area of their developmental power, as Drellich has also pointed out, and further consideration and expansion of this statement will be addressed later in this paper.

The actual issue of what the uterus functionally does in the female body, or its physiological role in the life cycle of women, has been strangely overlooked in psychoanalytic theorizing, possibly because most of the theorizers were men. This omission is probably even more a consequence of the mythic dimension of awe and wonder about life, a point raised by Bardwick in 1973.

Joseph Campbell in his writings stresses the importance of Otto Rank's construct of birth and by implication the uterus. To Rank the act of birth is an act of heroism; as the baby transforms itself from the intrauterine to an extrauterine, air-breathing creature. The uterus is consequently the organ that enobles.

Similarly Jung, borrowing from Eastern views of the male/ female universal principles, constructs his theories of the "Anima" archetype, i.e. of an omnipotent mother whose memory is present in the "collective unconscious."

Uterine function over the span of a woman's lifetime is seldom referred to as a factor in such theorizing. As Elizabeth Janeway pointed out in *Man's World, Woman's Place* (1971), there are few areas in social mythology that are free of man's fear of woman as earth mother, as all men must develop from women but never vice versa.

Since the unconscious is supposedly free of the dimensions of time, structuralist frameworks do not concern themselves with the difference between the significance of the uterus to a patient such as Freud's Dora or to a middle-aged woman such as myself. In Dora's dream the uterus was symbolized metaphorically by a treasure, a jewelry casket. It was in light of this universal metaphor, derived from a shared common human feeling, that my colleagues were reacting to my impending surgery. This universal symbol on a cognitive level would prove ultimately to be highly irrelevant to my current physical or emotional status (Freud 1901-1905, Volume 7).

I was NOT experiencing a great sense of loss as my own meditative and hypnagogic experiences would suggest. The treasure of the casket had long since been emptied, transformed into other, more intellectual forms, i.e. the uterus was now a vestigial organ. It was the experience of having been daughter, granddaughter, sister, lover, wife, female peer, mother and grandmother that translated into a development in personal growth. This growth bore fruit in my mind.

In 1980 Ethel Specter Person, upon reviewing attitudes to sexuality and sexual identity, stated that the contribution of object-relations theory to this field was the emphasis of the mother-child bond and the subsequent emergence of sensuality as part of core gender identity. This view shifts from the libido theory in the direction of the experiential and the interpersonal. Person speaks of gender identity as having various components, one of which she terms a "sex print," developmental sexual experience and sexual preference. She concludes as follows: "Many psychoanalytic theorists currently view sexuality as a motivational system which is derivative not from drive, but from the psychological sensual experience integrated through a series of object relations." Person continues: "One of the crucial differences between female and male sexuality is the invariable dependence of gender identity on sexuality in males, a dependence not invariably found in females."

Within a constricted format it is impossible to trace the development over the past 60 years towards the aforementioned viewpoint. I would have to review the work of Clara Thompson, Melanie Klein, Mary Jane Sherfey, Judith Bardwick, Ruth Moulton, Alexandra Symonds, Jean Baker Miller, Carol Gilligan and many others. I have selectively chosen and cited those sources which closely match my subjective and interpersonal experiences.

I parted from my uterus via a ruminative review of my personal female life track while my colleagues, those whose responses I detailed earlier, communicated with me out of a phallocentric, stereotypic paradigm which they still believe to be valid. We were, therefore, not really communicating. What I am sure was meant to be empathic was for me an additional burden.

Cognitive Approaches to Hysterectomy

Irving Bieber in his book *Cognitive Psychoanalysis* (1980) discusses organ ablation in general and hysterectomy in particular:

"Psychiatric reactions to organ ablation supervene under the following circumstances:

1. When there is significant diminution of self-esteem as a result of the ablation.

2. When there is interference in the individual's relatedness to other people.

3. When organ ablation either diminishes or eliminates a function which is important for the individual gratification of defensive adaptation, i.e., familiar, characterlogical ways of functioning."

There have been many studies in recent years, which bear out Bieber's statements. Gynecological, psychosomatic and nursing studies of hysterectomised women, done both prospectively and retrospectively between the years 1980-1998 stress the following findings:

1. Depression is the most common psychological condition encountered with regard to hysterectomy. It is more common in this surgical procedure than in many others, e.g., cholecystectomy. It is more common in dependent, traditionally oriented women, whose self esteem is based on their social value as a sex object or child bearer.

2. Nancy Roeske in a pioneer study of hysterectomy in 1980 concluded: " A hysterectomy does not produce significant psychopathology in a psychologi-

cally mature and healthy woman, i.e., there is a strong link between preoperative mental health and post-operative recovery, both physical and mental."

3. Vaginal procedures carry less risk for both pain and depression and should be done if at all possible (Kikku et al 1987). Most recently, laser surgery, surgery procedures such as laser ablation of the endometrium have been added to our surgical procedures. These may replace hysterectomy in younger women with severe menorrhagia. Thus, as technology advances, and there are more options for women to choose from, it becomes all the more important to reconsider our social and psychological myths in light of anachronistic and harmful, irrational attitudes. (Internet: http://www.mayohealth.org/mayo/9406/htm/myth sb. html, "Hysterectomy - It Can Be A Blessing But Alternatives Offer Choices: Myths Vs. Facts." Mayo Health O@sis 1996 Mayo Foundation for Medical Education and Research: Alexander, D., Atherton, Naji A., Pinion, S., Mollison, J., et al.: http://canada.silverplate.com/physicians/digest/abstract/abst28.htm, "Does Endometrial Ablation Cause Fewer Psychological Problems Than Hysterectomy?" "British Medical Journal" 1996; 312:280-284.)

4. Fantasies about the uterus, ovaries and sexual organs are reawakened by the impending surgery and by the surgery itself. These may be of a regressive, childhood nature, or as in my own case, vehicles for mourning and detachment from a body part about to be lost. In an early study in 1958, Drellich and Bieber worked with 23 hysterectomised women on the attitude to their reproductive organs. They found, "that patients who had here-

tofore never consciously formulated their attitudes towards a particular organ of their body, became aware that they harbored within themselves certain definite beliefs about their anatomy, their physiology and the value of a particular organ in their life adjustment. Some of these attitudes were undoubtedly the product of the phallocentric over-emphasis on what was then perceived as femininity."

5. Recent studies from the nursing field particularly stress the importance of a non male-dominated environment as important in both the pre- and post-operative periods. They stress the value of education, social support and collaboration between all care givers, including the empathic concern of the surgeon (Webb 1986). In the past, the feeling of being damaged goods after hysterectomy often led to depression. In a recent paper on young women who had been incest victims, O'Brien wrote about their seriously compromised sense of self. "Will he know about me?" was a question they asked themselves in later heterosexual relationships. In a parallel manner, a hysterectomized woman can be made to feel intruded upon and "taken from" by an uncaring and noncommunicative surgeon, with a similar feeling of a "damaged self" as a result.

6. There is need for the education of the public and the patient about hysterectomy and other related procedures. Despite the mass media and popular journal studies, it is indicated that the best absorbed knowledge is that which is imparted orally by the doctor or his assistant (Webb 1884, 1985) (Young 1995). In this

regard, the psychotherapist can also play a major role. Personality assessment and risk for depression or neurosis can be discussed and dealt with preoperatively. One might conduct the maintenance of therapy and psychopharmacology while hospitalized, or post-operatively if necessary, with some patients.

7. It takes anywhere between three months to three years for the process of mourning and readjustment to complete itself after hysterectomy. This time can be an opportunity for the development of pathology or of further personal growth. As such, it is a good time to institute therapy for those who wish it (Roeske 1980).

8. There is a lack of studies on the psychological meaning of hysterectomy in the different stages of the female life cycle. Clearly, a hysterectomy performed on a young woman of childbearing age is not the same as one done late in life on a middle-aged woman who is a grandmother or one who is middle- aged and never bore children. Drellich and Bieber mentioned guilt and a fear of punishment as a central dynamic in their 1958 patients. Studies done in the 1970s and 1980s do not mention this as much but concentrate instead on conflicts between gender and personhood roles. This is in keeping with social changes during the past 40 years but this does require further exploration.

The above summary of cognitive approaches to hysterectomy includes cross-cultutral studies from several countries East and West. The research data appears to be uniform and transculturally similar (Kikku 1987, Lalinec-Michaud 1984, 1985, Singh, et. al., 1983).

It is only when we collect more of the cognitive answers that we will be able to return to our mythologies and theories about female identity and the female reproductive organs and see which metaphors best fit the actual clinical female subjective experience. It is only out of such carefully documented experiences that a non-phallocentric theory about women's gender identity can emerge.

BIBLIOGRAPHY

Alexander, D., Atherton, Naji., Pinion, S., Mollison, J., et al: http// canada.silverplatter.com/ physicians/ digest/ abstract/ abst28.htm

"Does Endometrial Ablation Cause Fewer Psychological Problems Than Hysterectomy?" *British Medical Journal* 1996, 312:280-284.

Bieber, Irving: *Cognitive Psychoanalysis,* 1980. Ch. 15, pages 272-294. Jason   Aronson, New York.

Bardwick, Judith M.: *Psychology of Women,* 1971. Harper and Row, New York.

Campbell, Joseph and Moyers, Bill: *The Power of Myth,* 1988. Pages 1213-163, Doubleday, New York.

Cutler, Winifred: *Hysterectomy, Before and After,* 1988. Harper and Row, New York.

Drellich, Marvin: *Enduring Psychoanalytic Concepts of Female Psychology.* In "Changing Concepts in Psychoanalysis, " 1981. Ed. Sheila Klebanow. Gardner Press, New York.

Drellich, Marvin and Bieber, Irving et al: *The Psychological Impact of Cancer and Cancer Surgery*, 1956. "Cancer," Vol. 9, #6. Nov-Dec 1956. Pages 1, 120-1, 126. J.B. Lippincott and Co., New York.

Drellich, Marvin and Bieber, Irving: "The Psychological Importance of the Uterus and Its Functions," 1958. *The Journal of Nervous and Mental Disease*, Vol. 126, #4, April 1958.

Dorpat, T.L.: "Phantom Sensation of Internal Organs," 1971: *Comprehensive Psychiatry*, Jan. 1987, Pages 53-57.

Douglas, C.J. and Druss, R.G. "Denial of Illness: A Reappraisal," 1987. *General Hospital Psychiatry*, Jan. 1987, Pages 53-57.

Freud, Sigmund: "Fragment of an Analysis of a Case of Hysteria," *Standard Edition*, Vol. 7, 1901-1905, Pages 64-94. Hogarth Press, London.
Gjevik, Susan: "Your Health: Is Hysterectomy Necessary?," *Modern Maturity*, Feb-March 1989, Pg. 18.

Goldstein, M.Z.: "Aspects of Gender and Ethic Identity in Menopause," *Journal of American Academic Psychoanalysis*, Vol. 15, #3, July 1989, Pgs. 383-394.

Gould, D. and Wilson, Barnett J.: "A Comparison of Recovery Following Hysterectomy and Major Cardiac Surgery," *Journal of Advanced Nursing*, July 1985, Vol. #4, Pgs. 315-323.

Internet: http://www.mayohealth.org/mayo/9406/ htm/myth sb.html "Hysterectomy - It Can Be A Blessing But... To Hysterectomy Depend On Your Symptoms." Mayo Health O@sis 1996 Mayo Foundation for Medical Education and Research.

Internet: http://www.mayohealth.org/mayo/9406/ htm/myth sb.html "Hysterectomy - It Can Be A Blessing But Alternatives Offer Choices: Myths Vs.Facts." Mayo Health O@sis 1996 Mayo Foundation for Medical Education and Research.

Internet: http://www.nejm.org/public/1997/0336/ 0004/0290/1.htm "Alternative Techniques of Hysterectomy," *The New England Journal of Medicine*, January 23, 1997, Vol. 336 #4.

Internet: http://www.nih.gov/grants/guide/pa-files/PA-95-020.html "Decision Making Process in Women's Health." NIH Guide, Vol. 24, #1, January 13, 1995.
Internet: http://www.nih.gov/grants/guide/rfa-files/RFA-HS-96-002.html "MedTep Research On Non-Cancerous Uterine Conditions." NIH Guide, Vol. 25, #6, March 1, 1996.

Jones, Ernest: "The Early Development of Female Sexuality," in *Papers on Psychoanalysis*, Balliere, Tindall and Cox, London, 1950.

Janeway, Elizabeth: *Man's World, Woman's Place*, William Morrow and Co., 1971, New York.

Kikku, P. Lethinen, V. et al: "Abdominal Hysterectomy Versus Surpavaginal Uterine Amputation: Psychic Factors," *Ann, Chir. Gynecol (Supp) (Finalnd)*, 1987, Pgs. 6 - 2 7 , Subfile Index Medicus.

Kernberg, Otto: *Object Relations Theory and Clinical Psychoanalysis*, 1976, Ch. 9, Pgs. 241-275, Jason Aronson, New York.

Lalinec-Michaud and Engelsman, F.: "Depression and Hysterectomy, A Prospective Study," *Psychosomatics*, July 1984, Vol. 25, #7, Pgs. 550-558.

Lalinec-Michaud and Engelsman, F.: "Anxiety, Fears and Depression Related to Hysterectomy," *Can. J. Psych*, Feb 1985, Vol. 30, #1, Pgs. 22-47.

Luria, A. R.: *The Working Brain*, 1973, Chapter 1, Pgs. 19-99, Basic Books, New York. Newell, Linda: http:/ / web.ukonline.co.uk./ linda.newell/ associate/ discuss/ htm "CHOICES - The Hysterectomy Association's Discussion List." Choices@coolist.com, 1997 The Hysterectomy Association, Last update April 14, 1998.

Newton, N., Baron, E.: "Reactions to Hysterectomy; Fact or Fiction?" *Primary Care*, 1976, Pgs. 781-801, W.B. Saunders, Philadelphia, PA.

O'Brien, J.D.: "The Effects of Incest on Female Adolescent Development," *Journal of American Academy of Psychoanalysis*, 1987, Vol. 15, #1, Pgs. 83-93.

Person, Ethel Spector: "Sexuality as the Mainstay of Identity; Psychoanalytic Perspectives, " in *Women, Sex and Sexuality*, Ed: Catherine Stimpson and Ethel Spector Person, 1980, Pgs. 36-62, Chicago University Press.

Reiser, Morton: *Mind, Brain, Body*, 1980, Chapter 12, Pgs. 140-157, Basic Books, New York.

Roeske, Nancy: "Hysterectomy and Other Gynecological Surgeries, " in *The Woman Patient*, Vol. 1, Ed: M. Notman and C. Nadelson, 1980, Chapter 16, Pgs. 213-33, Plenum Press, New York.

Salter, J.R.: "Gynecological Symptoms and Psychological Distress in Potential Hysterectomy Patients, " *J. Psychosom. Res.*, 1985, Vol. 29, #2, Subfile Index Medicus.

Sandberg, S.I., Barnes, B.A., et al.: "Elective Hysterectomy: Benefits, Risks and Costs," *Med. Care*, Sept 1985, Vol 23, #9, Pgs. 1,067-1,085.

Singh, B., Raphael, B. et al.: "Post-Hysterectomy Adaptation: A Review and Report of Two Follow-Up Studies,

" Aust. N. Journ. of Psychiatry, Sept 1983, Vol 17, #3, Pgs. 227-235.

Toaff, Michael E.: http:// www.netreach.net/ - hysterectomyedu/ articles.htm   Alternatives to Hysterectomy"
1. One woman's decision against hysterectomy, by Natalie Angier, *New York Times*, Science section, February 18, 1977
2. "A Surgeon Specializes in Saving Wombs", by Nancy V. Greene, Main Line Times, Vol.67,#32, June 5, 1997 (published in Ardmore, PA)
3. "She Surfed to A Second Opinion," by Jo Cavallo, *Family Circle*, Computers Made Easy, Holiday edition, 1997
4. "Just Say 'Wait a Minute' ", by Cathy Perlmuter and Toby Hanlon, *Prevention*, January 1998.

Toaff, Michael E.: http:// www.netreach.net/ - hysterectomyedu/ myomecto.htm "Alternatives to Hysterectomy: Myomectomy"

Toaff, Michael E.: http:// www.netreach.net/ - hysterectomyedu/ whywould.htm "Why Would A Woman Resist Hysterectomy?"

Young, L., Humphrey, M.: "Cognitive Methods of Preparing Women for Hysterectomy: Does a Booklet Help?," *Br. Journ. Clin. Psychol.*, Nov 1985, Vol. 24, #4, Pgs. 303-304

Webb, C., Wilson, Barrett J.: "Hysterectomy: A Study in Coping with Recovery," *Journal Adv. Nurs.*, July 1983, Vol. 8, #4, Pgs. 311-319

Webb, C.: "Feminist Methodology in Nursing Research," *Journal Adv. Nurs.*, May 1984, Vol. 9, #3, Pgs. 249-256.

Webb, C.: "Professional, Lay and Social Support for Hysterectomy Patients," *Journal Adv. Nurs.*, March 1986, Vol. 11, #2, Pgs. 167-177.

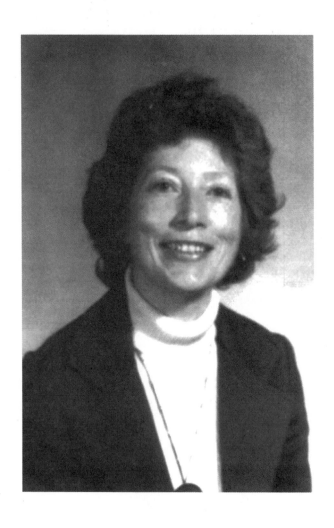

Opal W. Broner, Ph.D.

THE PSYCHOANALYTIC SIGNIFICANCE OF HYSTERECTOMY

Opal W. Broner, Ph.D.

We can all thank Dr. Davidson for her willingness to challenge dogma and tradition by examining the reality of her own experience. Her conclusions were well vindicated when the Science Section of the *New York Times* featured an article on a number of recent European studies with the headline, "Wide Beliefs On Depression In Women Contradicted." Daniel Goleman was reporting on a review in the *American Journal of Psychiatry* which stated that studies in England and other European countries found that not only were beliefs about negative emotional reactions to hysterectomy not substantiated, but that, "women who were depressed before a hysterectomy often recover from the depression after the operation." These reports are "little noted" in America, states Goleman, although he says, "A widespread belief among health professionals in America is that women who have hysterectomies are especially vulnerable to depression afterward." Furthermore, he reported that common beliefs about postpartum depression and depression at menopause were known to have no basis. These depressions, when occurring, were actually more related to marital conflict and other emotional stresses.

In my own reading and discussions, I have noted that many health professionals view hysterectomy as a likely prelude to a serious loss of libido and self esteem and to depression. How did these beliefs begin? What is their meaning? Were these beliefs perhaps more true in the past than at present, and if so why?

Dr. Davidson provides one clue when she refers to the positive transference that she developed toward her surgeon. The transference was necessary for subduing the fear that impending surgery incurs. She is a sophisticated and discerning individual. We can assume that Dr. Davidson's transference was tempered by objectivity as well as by her knowledge of her needs. For the average, less sophisticated woman, the transference could well bring about the fulfillment of the surgeon's concerns and expectations. The patient becomes severely depressed after surgery as the surgeon had anticipated. By contrast if the patient has a surgeon whose outlook for woman past childbearing is a casual "What do you need it for?", she is likely to feel resentful and misunderstood.

Dr. Davidson's characterization of her surgeon as a "realistic and caring person who would not unnecessarily mutilate my body or alternatively, not do enough to alleviate my discomfort," shows her awareness of the pitfalls which can be created by the personality and beliefs of the doctor. The mythic aspects of these beliefs - widely held, often unconsciously - can be found in anthropological and psychoanalytic writings. The mystique of the uterus, ideas of its function and value, has its foundation in the historical past. From biblical times through the present , women have been valued principally for their reproductive function. The uterus was perceived as a container where the "seed" - from the male - was planted, to grow and to flourish if "fertile" or to perish if the container was "barren." Men would consequently view a woman with a "dysfunctional" uterus (or a woman without a uterus) as of little value. Under such conditions, small wonder that a menopausal or hysterectomized woman would be depressed!

The Greeks attributed emotionalism (considered to be lacking in men and prominent in women) to dysfunctions of the uterus (hence, "hysteria). One hundred years ago hysterectomy and ovariectomy were common treatments for "excessive sexuality" (with, I suppose, a "normalizing" effect on the patient's personality and emotions). Throughout history, superstitions and cultural values have determined opinions about the uterus and its functions.

Medical, sociological and psychological research has contributed much knowledge since these earlier times. That knowledge can, however, be tainted by the unconscious residue of older beliefs and fears.

Presently women are urged to be sexual beings and not only in a reproductive capacity. Women are encouraged to be more than reproductive vessels and nurturers and even to be something other than these. Many young women are choosing not to have children for ethical or personal reasons. Dr. Davidson's gynagogic image of the fairy-like being emerging from her cervix, which she understood to represent her "brain children," is a lovely allegorical statement of how creative productions satisfy. In the past, however, the "brain children" of women were considered to be illegitimate outcasts, deformed and shunned by society. "Brain children" were often hidden away as were living children who were in some way imperfect. Virginia Woolf, in *A Room of One's Own* poignantly described the fate of a number of such "brain children" and of the women who created them in the past. Even today there is a tendency to denigrate women's artistic production. It is human reproduction, formed in cooperation with the male, not artistic production that is admired.

In the psychoanalytic sphere, Freud's symbolism of women's reproductive organs, inclusive of the metaphoric "jewel box", reflects the high value we place consciously and unconsciously on these organs. One of my patients, a woman in her 50s, dreamed that she came into a hotel room and saw cheap jewelry pasted on the walls. In her dream she looked in her jewelry box and noted that everything of value was gone. My patient had a "sinking feeling" that her husband would enter the room and upbraid her for having been careless with her jewels. This women had never had a hysterectomy but recently was separated from her husband and felt estranged from her children. The jewelry box and the hotel room represented the impermanence of the intimate ties in her life and her sense of loss of sexual attractiveness (she has had a breast augmentation and a facelift since her separation from her husband).

Ferenczi's notion of the centrality of the uterus in sexuality is a more extreme view. Horney describes it thus:

"...the real incitement to coitus, its true, ultimate meaning for both sexes, is to be sought in the desire to return to the mother's womb. During a period of contest, men acquired the privilege of really penetrating once more, by means of their genital organ, into a uterus. The woman, who was...in the subordinate position, was obliged to adapt her organization to this organic situation as was provided with certain compensations. She had to "content herself" with substitutes in the nature of fantasy and above all with harboring a child, whose bliss she shares. At the most, it is only in the act of birth that she perhaps has potentialities of pleasure denied to the man." (Horney, p. 59). In this scheme, not only does the woman find herself a passive instrument of the man's pleasure, but the woman without a uterus would even lack the ability to satisfy a man sexually because of his unconscious goals.

Horney, on the other hand, sees in the almost universal depreciation of women by males, an intellectual sublimation of an "intense envy of pregnancy, childbirth, and motherhood." (Horney, p. 60)

Somewhat more recently, Erikson's studies of pubescent girls and boys led him to postulate the female experience as being organized around "inner space" - the girls' fantasies tended to take place in protected interiors or

enclosed spaces, in contrast to the boys', which were intrusive and happening in the outdoors. While he does
not address directly the experience of hysterectomy, he
had vivid words to describe the grief of "emptiness" in
women:

"...Clinical observation suggests that in female experiences an 'inner space' is at the center of despair even as it
is the very center of potential fulfillment. Emptiness is the
female form of perdition - known at times to men of the
inner life - but standard experience for all women. To be
left, for her, means to be left empty, to be drained of the
blood of the body, the warmth of the heart, the sap of life.
How a woman thus can be hurt in depth is a wonder to
many a man, and it can arouse both his empathic horror
and his refusal to understand. Such hurt can be re-expe-
rienced in each menstruation, it is a crying to heaven in
the mourning over a child, and it becomes a permanent
scar in menopause. Clinically, this 'void' is so obvious that
generations of clinicians must have had a special reason
for not focusing on it. Maybe, even as primitive men
banned it with phobic avoidances and magic rituals of pu-
rification, the enlightened men of a civilization pervaded
by technological pride could meet it only with the interpretation that suffering woman wanted above all what
man had, namely, exterior equipment and traditional access to 'outer space.' " (Erikson, p.278)

Erikson's conclusions were based on his research and
clinical experience, but unavoidably influenced by the "selective attention" and "selective inattention" all of us fall
prey to. While I believe (coming from my own experience

and belief system) that he has pointed out an important truth. I concurrently believe that he has over generalized and has not taken into account the various life circumstances that affect women's reaction to, for example, menstruation and menopause.

Reviewing the research on the psychological side effects of hysterectomy, a brief study reveals few well-designed or unbiased studies. Most of the studies were conducted via questionnaires given out by doctors who performed the hysterectomy or who referred the patient to gynecologists who then did the surgery. Widely quoted is an investigation by D. H. Richards, an English general practitioner who found that 70% of his hysterectomy patients, as compared to 30% of women having other surgery, became depressed within three years of surgery. "Nearly 70% also suffered hot flashes, whether or not their ovaries had been removed, as well as urinary symptoms and extreme tiredness. Approximately half of the women had headaches, dizziness or insomnia. Women who had hysterectomies required one year to recover, while women who had other operations needed only three months to recuperate. Depression was most common in women who had their hysterectomies before the age of 40. (Payer, p. 23; also see Morgan, p. 222-223)

One writer states that, "Despite the assurances of most doctor-written books, that a well-adjusted woman should have no problems, several studies that have attempted to follow up women after their hysterectomies have shown a high rate of depression and other psychiatric illness." She cites a study by N. Kaltreider, a psychiatrist at Langley Porter Institute (UCSF) which researched women under 40 who had undergone hysterectomy for reasons other than cancer, "About 60% of these women were suffering a degree of altered self-image, depression and other symptoms." An Israeli study is also cited, showing that "nearly half" of patients showed "depression, loss of libido, or various physical symptoms following hysterectomy." (Payer, p. 24)

In contrast, American gynecologist B. C. Richards, conducted a survey of 340 of his patients who had hysterectomies in 1975, and 90% of them responded that they were pleased with their surgery and felt better or somewhat better than before. (Morgan, p. 220-221

More relevant to psychoanalytic implications was a study published in 1958 by M. Drellich and I. Bieber, also referred to in Dr. Davidson's paper. Drellich and Bieber interviewed at length 23 patients who were to have hysterectomies (1) before the operation, (2) during their hospital stay and (3) in a 6-12 month follow up. The focus rather than being on the symptoms was on other feelings about the hysterectomies and its meaning for them. As might be expected, "for some women, even though they desired no more children, the knowledge that they were able to bear children gave them the feeling of being complete and feminine. The loss of childbearing ability was viewed as rendering a woman something less than a complete female." (Drellich and Bieber, 1958). The cessation of menstruation was also viewed a loss by many of those interviewed, who saw, for example, "the monthly cycle as a part of the rhythm of life." Others felt the uterus to be a source of strength and health. One 40 year old patient clearly illustrated her concept to the uterus as her sex organ. She consciously visualized her uterus as having the characteristics of an "internal penis". She felt that the intermittent distention of her abdomen was caused by her uterus becoming swollen and erect due to sexual desire. Because of her husband's indifference to her sexual needs and her reluctance to seek an alternative sexual outlet, she felt that her uterus remained engorged and turgid, allegedly returning to normal only after her infrequent sexual intercourse with her husband. She stated, "If I were a man, I'd be walking around with a big penis all the time."

Drellich and Bieber also found that several of the women felt the hysterectomy, or the disease which necessitated it, to be a punishment for past transgressions for which they felt guilty.

At the other extreme, W. Gifford-Jones, a Canadian gynecologist, writes of the apparently not uncommon phenomenon of women who talk their doctors into performing hysterectomies. Although he tends to attribute this predominantly to an "instant cure philosophy" for every ailment or discomfort, it would be interesting to know more about the unconscious motivations of these women.

Other studies (e.g., Barker, 1968; Meikle, Stewart, et al, 1977; Patterson and Craig, 1963; Roeske, 1978 and a review by Niles Newton, 1976) conclude that physical and psychological sequelae of hysterectomy depend greatly upon the previous psychiatric history of the patient, the symbolic meaning to the patient, the attitude of the doctor and of the patient's family (especially the husband), the age of the woman, her basic physical condition, her general attitude toward surgery and the patients own security in her own feminine identity.

In sum, the emotional outcome of a hysterectomy, while strongly affected by both the conscious and unconscious significance to the patient, does not seem to be universal or uniform. Even when the loss of the uterus is mourned by the woman as the loss of a significant component of her body and her history, and if she is young, as the relinquishing of hope of motherhood, the uterus in most cases does not seem to be the core of feminine identity. Psychoanalytic theory must take this into account in revising the present phallocentric ideas about female psychology.

BIBLIOGRAPHY

Barker, M. C. "Psychiatric Illness After Hysterectomy, " (1968) *British Medical Journal Vol. II*, Pages 91-95 (In Morgan, op. cit.).

Drellich, M. and Bieber, I. "The Psychological Importance of the Uterus and Its Functions", (1958), in *Journal of Mental and Nervous Diseases*, #126:1, Pages 322-336.

Erikson, Erik H. "Identity, Youth and Crisis", (1968) New York, W.W. Norton and Co., *Austen Riggs Monograph #7*, Page 278.

Ferencizi, S. *Versuch Einer Genitaltheorie*, (1924), in Horney, op. cit.

Gifford-Jones, W. *What Every Woman Should Know*, (1977). Funk and Wagnalls, New York, Pages 71-72 and 149-150.

Goleman, D. Beliefs on "Depression in Women Contradicted." *New York Times*, January 9, 1990, Page 1, Section C.

Horney, Karen *Feminine Psychology,* (1967). New York, W.W. Norton & Co.

Meikle, Stewart, et al. *An Investigation into the Psychological Effects of Hysterectomy,* (1977). In *Journal of Mental and Nervous Diseases,* #164:1, Page 36.

Morgan, Susanne *Coping With Hysterectomy,* (1982). New York, Dial Press.

Newton, N. and Baron, E. "Misconceptions Concerning The Psychological Effects of Hysterectomy," (1976). *American Journal of Obstetrics and Gynecology,* 85:1, Page 104

Patterson, R.M. and Craig, J.B. "Misconceptions Concerning the Psychological Effects of Hysterectomy," (1963). *American Journal of Obstetrics and Gynecology,* 85:1, Page 104

Richards, Bruce "Hysterectomy: From Women to Women," (1978). *American Journal of Obstetrics and Gynecology,* 131:4, Pages 446-452

Richards, D.H. *Depression After Hysterectomy,* (1973). *The Lancet,* August 25, 1973, Pages 430-433. In Morgan, op. cit. and Payer, op. cit. (1974), *A Post-Hysterectomy Syndrome, The Lancet,* October 26, 1974, in Morgan, op. cit. and Payer, op. cit.

Payer, Lynn *How to Avoid A Hysterectomy*, (1987). New York, Pantheon Books.

Roeske, N.C. *Quality of Life and Factors Affecting the Response to Hysterectomy*, (1978). J. Family Practice, 7:3, Pages 483-488

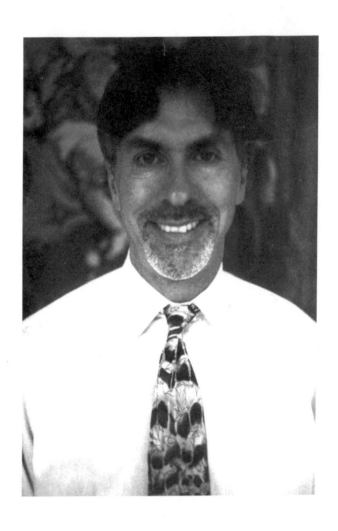

Steven Lesk, M.D.

CANCER: A PERSONAL PERSPECTIVE

Steven Lesk, M.D.

Cancer is an illness from which there is no cure, only relative degrees of well-being. A multi-dimensional affliction, it renders its victims physically, emotionally and psychosocially scarred. The social stigmata of the illness is often as devastating as the somatic. There is, however, much to be gained from the cancer experience provided one survives it. These benefits include a sharpening of perspective, a heightened sense of concern for one's physical and mental health, a greater appreciation of life and an enhancement of spiritual values. It may free one from the more mundane, neurotic concerns of daily living while centering one's attention on the realistic perils of existence.

This paper draws on my personal experience with testicular cancer. With this as a foundation, I would like to portray as accurate a picture as possible of the cancer experience. There are a multitude of approaches to the subject, not all of which can be touched upon here. For example, one might consider theories on the psychosocial etiology of cancer, the role of stress and depression, the impact of the diagnosis on the patient and family, coping skills required to endure the experience, etc.

In May of 1988 I presented a paper before the American Academy of Psychoanalysis on the implications of modern psycho-oncology research for psychoanalysis (Lesk, 1988). In it I pointed to research suggesting that states of mind have a bearing on both the onset and prognosis of cancer. I even proposed that psychoanalytic therapy might have a role in the prevention of the disease, possibly a role in prolongation of survival, and most certainly in enhancing the quality of life and coping skills of the cancer sufferer. This remains a fascinating area of ongoing study.

In this paper I would like to focus on the experiential world of the cancer victor. I will first concentrate on my own illness, then review some of the literature on cancer patients and later explore the psychoanalytic implications of the disease and its treatment as well as the broader picture of the health care system's approach to the person who suffers this catastrophe. Reorientation to a cancer phobic world will be examined, including my own personal coping strategies. Ultimately I would like to mention many of the positives in the cancer journey and what the individual and society might do to promote adaption.

My Testicular Cancer

I was fortunate to keep a journal of my illness experience. I recommend this to all who must endure an illness for both therapeutic and practical reasons. One tends to forget the details of the ordeal which may be important for later consultation.

On Thursday, January 3rd, 1985, a mass was discovered in my right testicle. Since it had appeared so suddenly I doubted that it could be a tumor but as a physician I knew that a suspicious testicular lesion had to be investigated. Tuesday in a urologist's office I trembled with the news that my right testicle had to be removed and that chemotherapy and further surgery were less than remote possibilities. My wife and I canceled a scheduled visit with her sister, shared tears and gathered our mental forces for the ensuing struggle.

I chose to tell only those at work who needed to know and made an excuse for my absence to the rest of my team. Patients were advised that I had a sudden vacation. To this day I continue in the workplace to reveal only the minimum about my cancer. This information is never volunteered.

I obtained a second opinion which confirmed the probable diagnosis of cancer and the appropriateness of the proposed treatment plan. I was scheduled for admission to the hospital on January 15, 1986. Fantasies of tumor cells breaking off from the primary plagued my waiting days. I attributed every ache and pain to metastases. On admission day we were called blessedly early by the hospital only to be told that no beds were available. As luck would have it, the heating system in our apartment failed. We were confined in a cold apartment awaiting salvation. The only relief was a trip to our attorney's warm office to sign a will. The next day we were finally allowed to come to the hospital to await eventual admission to the urology ward.

My anxiety level ascended to new heights as I contemplated surgery. I was very fortunate to be in psychoanalysis at the time. My analyst agreed to visit me in the hospital. This is a luxury that should be pursued, if at all possible, by all patients.

The surgery went smoothly. The surgeon announced that the tumor was malignant and that further tests were required to determine the next course of action. These tests included a CAT scan of the abdomen and pelvis, tomograms of the lungs and tumor marker studies. I recall vividly my reaction to the inclusion of tomograms to the stipulated tests. No explanation had been given and I sensed that the end was near.

Both my human chorionic gonadotropin (HCG) and alpha-fetoprotein (AFP), indices of tumor activity, were elevated. The HCG and AFP should have returned to normal if all the cancer cells had been excised. In addition my right breast was noticeably enlarged. Consideration was given to a lymphangiogram, not routinely done at this phase of treatment. Getting information was similar to finding water in an oasis. Each drop was precious. I learned more from the oncologist who was called in as a consultant than I did from my surgeon or his partner, kamikaze pilots, who sailed in and out of my room, ready to drop their deadly but eagerly awaited cargo.

My relationship with my surgeon was open enough for him to help me to find expert follow-up care. I was surprised, however, that I was never offered specific counseling addressing cancer. No one offered me cancer support group numbers. There was no effort made to put me in touch with other cancer patients, to find out how I was contending with cancer or to offer my wife and family support and information. I found out independently where the nearest and best cancer center was and some names affiliated with this center.

I was discharged on January 26 when it was determined that all my test results were negative, including a substantial drop in tumor markers. My diagnosis was non-seminomatous germ cell of the testicle, treated with orchiectomy alone and with no evidence of spread. My next task was to transfer my case to a nearby cancer center and prepare to return to work. The center had accepted my case and offered me participation in a study of stage one tumors treated with observation alone through CAT scans every eight weeks and monthly tumor markers and chest x-rays. The alternative was to opt immediately for the retro-peritoneal lymph node dissection with a potential side effect of retrograde ejaculation. To aid in the decision, a lymphangiogram was scheduled.

Throughout my hospitalization my saving grace was the support system which swarmed around me, a support system headed by my wife of only seven months Eileen. My parents, therapist, assorted relatives, friends and co-workers supplemented my "team". Cancer patients lacking such a team are severely handicapped. I had never been so grateful to have them around. Stress was, however, obvious in the faces of those close to me and my own anxiety level was astronomic. Many of my actions and decisions became robotic in nature. Logical thinking was diminished. This state, existing with a support network, would have been terrible if confronted in an isolated position. I was also extremely fortunate to have the financial and insurance coverage needed to avoid disaster. I shudder to think of what cancer represents for those less fortunate.

I met with an internationally known expert who was to assume my follow-up care. He presented the pros and cons of surgery versus exclusively observation. The lymphangiogram had gone smoothly. I was impressed with the competence and caring of the nurse who threaded a thin catheter into a lymphatic vessel in my right great and second toes. The results were negative, suggesting that the lymph nodes were clean.

After agonizing endlessly over the issue of aftercare and receiving advice, both solicited and unsolicited, from numerous people, I agreed to participate in the study protocol. Being able to help others who would be afflicted in the future was a reward in itself. I worried about the x-radiation but contended with it to avoid the possibility of sterility. My wife and I still dreamed of having a family. We were informed that only 20% of patients in my position had a recurrence.

I entered into an extended period of routine cancer follow-ups. I endured monthly and then bimonthly chest x-rays, tumor marker studies and CAT scans. The concept of recurrence was unimaginable, not within our grasp. Each return visit was further evidence that the tumor had been completely excised. Both my HCG and AFP levels remained down except for slight aberrations which proved repeatedly to be false alarms. My journal entries became increasingly infrequent. My therapy helped me put the experience behind me and to perceive it as another incident within the framework of life. January of 1986 we held a large family party to celebrate my continued good health and my passing of the Psychiatry and Neurology boards.

On April 7, 1986 my wife received a frightening phone call. She called me at work, crying that the cancer center wanted me to return because the latest scan had revealed two enlarged nodes. I was aware of some lymph node enlargement appearing on the scan, had even indicated it to the urologist. Since the nodes were on the contralateral side from my original tumor, the chance of recurrence seemed minimal. I paged the urologist and reminded him of our previous conversation. He replied that our "famous expert" had reviewed the films and perceived the possibility of recurrence.

For convenience I had started getting my scans at the hospital where I worked. They had become as routine for me as blood tests are for others. Subsequent to my wife's call, I immediately scheduled an abdominal-pelvic scan. Eileen joined me while I sipped large quantities of orange-tasting contrast material to the point of nausea. My scan was delayed and I waited in nervous anticipation. I had earlier arranged for the chairman of the radiology department to interpret the film. He had neatly outlined and circled two enlarged nodes below the diaphragm. There could be no mistake about it; I was in for at least the surgery and probably chemotherapy.

On April 15, 1986 I underwent a retro-peritoneal lymph node dissection. I felt calm though the more accurate characterization was numb. I was asked to decide if I would have the first chemo in the hospital or recuperate at home for a month. My wife and her family gathered around me as if attending a wake. It was an interminable 8 hour wait. The news was excellent ; no cancer had been found. The reason for the lymph nodes' enlargement was not determined. The enlargement could be attributed to the radiation itself or some minor infection. I called it my "pseudo-recurrences". My recovery was painful but un-eventful. We underwent the stress of cancer recurrence but the end results were a blessing.

A Patient's Update

Ten years have elapsed since my second operation, The cancer experience is still vivid. Nothing can surpass the word cancer for its implied urgency, the fear it gener-ates and the resultant compelling call to action. The world stops. Everything becomes secondary to the all-pervasive desire to be rid of the cancer.

Studies indicate the families of cancer patients are as emotionally affected as the patients. My wife and I were married only seven months when the tumor was noticed. The cancer brought us closer, but for many cancer tends to separate and divide. We were fortunate and have contended successfully with the increased stress. There were certainly times of intense emotion and irritable intervals of waiting, decision making, etc., yet these strengthened our relation-ship. I recall several years of travel to Sloan-Kettering for follow-up examinations and blood tests. Prior to each visit everything was perceived negatively. After that same visit, with a broad sigh of relief, we would smile and laugh.

The apex of stress was experienced prior to my first surgery. We had expected admission to the hospital but discovered instead a lack of available beds. We called, waited and recalled. As we persisted in calling, the heat went out in our apartment. Our spirits flagged. We felt not only endangered but rejected.

Eileen, as the wife of a cancer "victor", has been understandably somewhat overprotective of me. She will occasionally think one of my breast areas has swollen, endemic to testicular cancer, and become very alarmed. She is very apprehensive about the emergence of any lump on my body, a prelude to the recurrence of cancer. Eileen urges me to lower my stress level, citing the relationship of excesses and increased risk. She has experienced and continues to experience an emotional whirlwind with me.

I have been irrevocably affected by my cancer battle. I am hypervigilant to signs and symptoms of disease. Every cough, sore throat, headache is a potential cancer threat. I see specialists when a symptom persists or has an unusual quality. This is a positive since I believe that prevention is the cure for cancer, but it can create its own anxieties.

I worry about toxins in the environment. I avoid situations where toxin exposure is possible or suspected. There was at one time a strange odor in my car. I was briefly convinced that it would imminently result in cancer. My life expectancy is viewed as foreshortened; though statistically within demographic parameters, it is the same anticipated span as that of someone who has never experienced cancer. I work out religiously, enjoying it, believing that it will stave off indefinitely the aging process. Diet is a constant concern. I have developed a bowel obstruction that is probably related to adhesions from my lymph node dissection. Twice I have been admitted to the hospital and once experienced the dreaded nasogastric tube. This may eventually require surgical correction. In the meantime I contend with a soft food only dietary regime.

Finally, there is a part of me that cannot forego belief in a psychodynamic etiology of cancer. There lingers a suspicion that cancer is a perverse manifestation of self-directed rage or the ultimate masochistic revenge - "I'll destroy myself before others get the chance to do me harm". This represents an expectation of harm which would emanate from superego conflicts. A mind which is so ready to punish success, especially success that surpasses one's father's, might choose cancer or mental illness or even suicide as the affliction du jour. This remains, however, a vague suspicion and a relic which I unearth in fragments.

Cancer has irrevocably altered my perspective on life, pain and suffering. Though I recognize the existence and seriousness of illnesses other than cancer, I do not perceive these illness to be as horrific as cancer. Even mental illness, however exquisite the suffering, is reduced in severity through comparison to cancer. The mental ward and the cancer ward are two very distinct environments. For me a nightmare would be realized in being a denizen of the latter rather than the former.

Pain and suffering are very real to me. It amazes me how many people suffer in silence, never acknowledged. Through the varied media we are acquainted with "great" people. Some of my heroes are confined to the wards, suffering but still praying for the continuation of life. Other heroes are the doctors and researchers who struggle daily to circumscribe terrible afflictions. Rarely are these heroes mentioned. They are reduced by television to two-dimensional characters limited by the scripts of maudlin dramas.

In a million ways I am oblivious as to how cancer has affected me. As a cancer patient I was forced to endure a great deal, but I endured only a fraction of what other patients did. It is these multitudes of people who desperately require help, reassurance and understanding. The studies that I've read all acknowledge the high rate of depression among cancer patients. Not once during my cancer journey did a mental health professional inquire as to my condition. There remains a phenomenal lack of involvement with cancer patients by mental health professionals. This is a great failure within the system. Can this pattern be altered, be corrected?

The Literature

The American Cancer Society (1990) lists cancer as the number two cause of death in this country. Number one is cardiovascular disease. While abdominal and uterine cancers demonstrated declining mortality rates between 1930 and 1986, lung cancer rates have continued to rise in both sexes (Silverberg, 1990). Testicular cancer afflicts 9.7 of every 100,000 men between the ages of 25 and 29. It is the most common form of cancer in men between the ages of 20 and 34 in the United States, according to del Regato, et al. (1985). There is a somewhat lower incidence among African-Americans. Testicular tumors evolve with minimal symptomology, often coming to attention only upon metastasizing to the retroperitoneum where lumbar pain or urinary obstruction may ensue (del Regato, et al., p. 711). Delay in seeking consultation may tragically result in retroperitoneal, lung or brain metastases as is seen in more extensive disease. More fortunate patients, including myself, upon noticing a fullness, swelling or weight in the testicle elicit further investigation.

Between the years 1960-1963, the five year testicular cancer survival rate for white males was 63%, by 1980-1985 it increased to 91%. This can largely be attributed to a combination chemotherapy of more extensive tumors with cisplatinum (Silverberg, 1990). Blandy, et al. (1983) state, "Today, we all expect that the young man who comes up with testicular cancer will be cured, and it has been seriously suggested that any death from testicular cancer should be made the object of a confidential enquiry similar to that which today regularly follows the unexpected death of a mother in pregnancy" (p. 209).

Themes in the Literature

Considerable scientific attention has been directed to the multidimensional effect of cancer on the individual. This subject is not readily amenable to rigorous scientific inquiry. Quality of life, as a concept, is nebulous enough to defy uniformity of approach. As described by de Haes and van Knippenberg (1985), quality of life is perceived either globally or in terms of specific criteria, either subjectively or objectively. These authors emphasized the relative lack of validated instruments and design approaches. Quigley (1989) commented on the relative lack of sensitivity of the instruments used to measure psychological distress in long-term survivors. The studied population is probably more attuned than most to the issue of the quality of life.

It is the anecdotal reports in their treatment of the cancer experience, that frequently add an extra dimension to and enhance pure research. Mack in 1984 and Green in 1987 in "The New England Journal of Medicine" as well as popular but tragic works by Gilda Radner (1989) and Jill Ireland (1987) highlight the importance of a reorganization of priorities and massive alterations in lifestyles, reflective of an increased awareness of the quality of life. Cancer is a mandate for personal change, augmenting the importance of each minute of life that remains.

It is, therefore, not surprising that some research indicates a more than satisfactory adjustment by cancer survivors (McMahon, 1987; Cassileth, et al., 1984) while other studies emphasize the subtle impairments in some cancer victors (Schmale, et al., 1983: Quigley, 1989: Ell, et al., 1989; Worden and Weisman, 1980). According to Ell et al (1989), "Although most patients improve from baseline measures of psychological distress, there is evidence that 20% to 30% of patients continue to experience clinically significant distress and poorer well-being long after diagnosis" (p. 406).

What is the degree of diagnosable mental illness among cancer patients? Studies are conflicting though most indicate a significant degree of clinical depression, anxiety and other disorders (Plumb and Holland, 1977; Derogatis, et al., 1983; Bukberg, et al., 1984; Silberfarb, 1984). Most diagnoses are in the realm of adjustment disorders. Major depression is, however, found in a significant percentage. Evans et al. (1988) discovered that 23% of patients, admitted to a gynecological tumor service, suffered from major depression. This study emphasized the importance of pharmacological treatment. Depression must be diagnosed primarily on the basis of non-somatic symptomatology since physical complaints may be secondary to the disease process. Psychosis is relatively rare. Derogatis et al. (1983) assessed 215 cancer patients and found 47% to have a DSM 1V diagnosis. This 47% could further be analyzed to be: 68% adjustment disorders, 13% major depressive disorders, 8% organic mental disorders, 7% personality disorders and 4% anxiety disorders.

Suicidal ideation was discovered in only a few of Peck's (1972) sample of 50 cancer patients. In contrast Breibert (1987) perceived suicide to be more prevalent among cancer patients than the general population. Those at greatest risk are those with the worst prognosis - experiencing depression, pain, delirium and loss of control. This high-risk group may have preexisting psychopathology, made prior suicide attempts and suffer from exhaustion and fatigue.

Is there a correlation between a psychiatric diagnosis or group of diagnoses and a greater incidence of cancer? Harris concluded that schizophrenics may be more prone to breast cancer and less prone to lung cancer for reasons unrelated to personal habits. As soon as the diagnosis is made, each patient surveys presumably causative risk factors, most of which may be irrational. The Western Electric study (Persky et al..1987) monitored over a period in excess of 20 years more than 2000 employees. It was discovered that "...depression as measured by the Minnesota Multiphasic Personality Inventory (MMPI) ...was positively associated with 20-year incidence and mortality from cancer" (p. 435).

After an exhaustive review of the literature, my own conclusion (Lesk, 1988) was that research points to several "Achilles' heels" related to cancer susceptibility. These "Achilles' Heels" include bereavement, personality traits emphasizing suppression of anger and emotions in general, a dysthymic stance and immune suppressing situations such as social isolation and extreme stress. Early childhood losses and lack of emotional closeness to parents are mentioned in other reviews and have been studied (Redd and Jacobsen, 1988). Greer et al. (1979) emphasized the importance of a "fighting spirit" in promoting survival in a series of breast cancer patients followed for ten years. Achterberg et al. (1977) believe that there are "...significant emotional aspects connected not only with the course of malignancy, but also with the onset of the disease" (p. 421). They encourage the development of therapeutic support systems designed to elicit these aspects. Spiegel et al. (1989) compared two matched groups of metastatic breast cancer patients. One group received a year of weekly group therapy and self hypnosis for pain; the other did not. After ten years of follow-up, the therapy group showed significantly longer survival. Peck (1972) presents patients who believe that their cancer is a punishment for some forbidden wish or longing. When this construct is clarified for them, they become less depressed and improve.

Theoretical issues aside, what do we know about the effects of cancer on the individual? Many do cope well, yet cancer has potentially devastating effects on all areas of patients' lives. Rieker et al. (1985) noted that their sample of testicular cancer indicated improved functioning in the areas of outlook on life, relationship with children, fear of death and self respect. The exceptions were those who had suffered impaired sexual functioning. Many of them continued to manifest psychological disturbances. Treatments which have side effects related to sexual dysfunction, mutilation and infertility are probably the most damaging psychologically. This fact has been underemphasized. Mutilating surgery with its castrating implications seems to wreak psychological havoc on many individuals. Such themes should be explored carefully. Mastectomy is very disturbing to some women. This fact should be ascertained prior to surgery (Dean, 1988). If these women are given the option of a less mutilating procedure, they may do better. Green (1987) could not locate any study on the psychological effects of orchiectomy. More research is required to determine which treatments convey the most emotional morbidity and the psychodynamic implications of different varieties of cancer.

Schmale et al. (1983) commented on the increased preoccupation with health status and the decreased sense of self-control in cancer victors. There is a sense among cancer patients that lightning has already struck once; they are cursed and more prone to catastrophes. Some have labeled the fear of recurrence the "Damocle's Syndrome" (Quigley, 1989). This fear is omnipresent and feeds into one's natural hypochondriasis. This state is particularly acute in the stage between diagnosis and surgery (Stam, et al., 1986). Every twinge is viewed as a metastasis, every headache a brain tumor. Many authors have commented on how stressful a recurrence can be (Silberfarb, et al., 1980; Fiore, 1979). This is a time when any denial as to the severity of an illness is shattered. Chronic treatments such as radiation or chemotherapy are particularly stressful (Wasserman, et al., 1987: Fiore, 1979).

Worden and Sobel (1978) found that patients with greater ego strength, as measured by Barron's ego strength scale, coped better with the cancer experience. This finding certainly is not surprising. What should be analyzed are the types of patients and the situations that are most conducive to psychological morbidity. The elderly seem to cope better with cancer (Holland and Massie, 1987). This could·be credited to a greater exposure to hospitals.

In addition to the obvious health concerns, cancer victors are plagued by financial, insurance and employment concerns. (Rieker, et al., 1985; Lansky, et al., 1986). Insurance companies are extraordinarily prejudiced against cancer victors. This prejudice is not mitigated by the available and very positive statistics. Government intervention would seem necessary. Many cancer patients do not discuss their illness. They fear job discrimination and social ostracism. This avoidance of conversation heightens and perpetuates their sense of isolation, isolation even from their families. Job mobility is frequently curtailed by a fear of exposing one's medical history.

We have some knowledge about the factors that promote successful adaption to cancer. Goodwin et al. (1987) found that, "Unmarried persons with cancer have decreased overall survival." Other authors have questioned this conclusion (Goldberg and Cullen, 1985). Illness can have a powerful effect on close relationships, strengthening or destroying them. Rieker et al. (1985) state, "...68% of the married men indicated that relationships with spouses were strengthened...whereas 74% of lover relationships were strained" (p. 1119). The husbands of breast cancer patients experienced distress equivalent to that of their spouses. This distress decreased over time (Northouse and Swain, 1987). Sexual functioning is a major determinant of a relationship's future. The benefits of family and psychosocial support are frequently mentioned in the literature (Kriesel, 1987; Allen, 1981; Spiegel, et al., 1981; Goldberg and Cullen, 1985). Goldberg and Cullen (1985) state that there is "...some evidence suggesting that individuals claiming religious affiliation cope better with cancer" (p. 805). They also mention the importance of previous death experiences. A physician's positive and hopeful demeanor and a good physician-patient relationship are viewed by many to be crucial coping elements (Siegel, 1989; Allen, 1981; Quigley, 1989; Kaufman, 1989).

248

In a study by Ell et al. (1989) of 253 newly diagnosed cancer patients, only 10% had seen a mental health worker and only 6% attended a post-diagnosis support group 9-12 months later. They stated, " These results are disturbing if they reflect lack of awareness of access to appropriate interventions rather than personal choice" (p. 412). Too few patients and families obtain needed psychosocial services. Rainey (1985) reported on his experience with the UCLA psychosocial cancer counseling line, which provided telephone counseling to cancer patients, families and other concerned parties. The most frequent request on the part of patients was for referrals to support groups. Interestingly, the most frequent calls from families concerned guidance in locating help. Anxiety about illness, concern about changing family roles and difficulties with physician-patient relationships were also frequent topics of concern. The need for therapeutic intervention is decidedly greater than the supply. The information about such services is not as readily available as it should be.

Not every patient wants or should receive counseling, although two-thirds of a group of newly-diagnosed, "at risk" for psychological disturbance cancer patients did accept counseling referrals. Worden and Weisman (1980) found a group of refusers who could not cope with any psychosocial intervention. They appeared threatened by the proposed treatment, interpreted it as a sign that their prognosis was poor and viewed the treatment as potentially disequilibrating. Nevertheless, the authors state, "Patients who at higher predicted risk receive intervention tend to have lower emotional distress scores from two to six months into their illness..." (p. 103) Certain patients need to wall off the experience of cancer, its threat to their masculinity and to their survival. Wellisch (1984) recommends groups that mix education and therapy. He views this approach as the least threatening. Fiore (1979) calls for a holistic approach. The patient is actively involved at every step in order to counteract the feeling of helplessness. Fiore also discussed the cancer patient's suggestibility and the secondary gain of having cancer. These two themes are often ignored.

Discussion

Cancer can be equated to psychoanalysis. If one survives either, it is a painful but enriching, growth-inducing experience. Cancer can be ego-enhancing. In psychodynamic terms, the super ego aligns with the ego as irrational guilt vanishes. Neuroses are abandoned in an effort to augment the ego's ability to navigate an often puzzling health care system. The individual learns a lesson in perspective, what is and is not very important. The id retreats in its primitive perception that interference with the ego at this point could result in annihilation. One learns to care more profoundly about oneself.

The grandiosity of the id is abandoned as mortality and vulnerability become more evident. The goodness of others is brought into sharper focus as family, friends and health care personnel are perceived as critical elements of patient support.

In light of the aforementioned the patient may view his cure as a return to a previous state of guilt and its dominance. He may secretly yearn for relapse as a means of re-empowering the ego, reexperiencing the mastery thrust upon it. It is here that psychoanalysis, psychotherapy, both group and individual, can be critical to the patient's forging of alliances with the super ego, maintaining a positive image of others through support systems and promoting the patient's ability to be genuinely concerned about himself.

I believe that serious illness should be approached as a sudden shift in the balance between the ego and the id, assisted by the super ego. The patient may spend the succeeding years haunted by his experience, attempting to recreate it.

Cancer research is vital and more is definitely required. The cancer journey is, however, a human process best understood through case histories and anecdotal reports. My own cancer shook me to the core and empowered me to move in many directions at once. During the period subsequent to my second surgery, I have changed jobs twice. One of those jobs was as acting chairman of a psychiatric department. My wife and I moved to the Midwest though we lacked any social contacts there. I have written a book about my experiences which I am attempting to publish. I am dabbling in an acting career. I have written and presented papers such as this. I have developed a keen interest in the psychosocial aspects of cancer.

My activities are all part of an ongoing effort to come to terms with my illness. I haven't yet made the treatment of cancer patients part of my professional focus. This is, however, a viable option for the future. At the very least, I would like to remain academically involved in the study of cancer and its ramifications. All of the aforementioned pursuits are creative ways in which I have attempted to cope with the experience of illness. Although I did not get involved with cancer support groups, my own therapy has been a partial substitute for this. Other positive effects of my experience have been a heightened sense of spirituality, concern for my physical health and that of others, exercise, meditation and a concerted effort to appreciate every day, or rather every minute, of my life.

In following the cancer trail, I was surprised and dismayed by many things. Cancer patients require more psychosocial interventions of all types. They should be encouraged to participate in some form of therapy while being given the option to decline. Perhaps because I am a psychiatrist, not one of my health care providers suggested any form of social intervention. I suspect, however, that most patients' experiences are similar. Too often families, if there are any, don't know how to help and cannot take the place of professional intervention or support groups.

Patients must be treated expeditiously once they are informed that they might have a malignancy, a recurrence or other complications in order to minimize irrational fears and concerns. I remember asking my oncologist if my headaches could be cerebral metastases. All patients have such concerns. Procedures need to be explained thoroughly and optimistically to patients to promote understanding and to foster hope. Patients should be encouraged to ask questions assertively and to take charge of those aspects of their treatment that they can reasonably be expected to assume.

Psychiatric consultations should be liberally available. Medical treatment for depression and anxiety should be more frequently employed. Concern for the dignity and preferences of terminal patients must be maintained, including adequate pain management. Health care workers must keep in mind the vulnerability, dependency and the plain suffering of the patient. Logical thinking under such circumstances can become very difficult for the patient.

Wish List for Cancer Patients

My recommendations to all those patients who must undergo the cancer experience are as follows:

1) Obtain therapy in one form or another, including self-help or support groups, individual or group private treatment, etc. Studies now suggest that this may protract survival time. Therapy will most certainly improve the quality of your life;

2) Get the best medical treatment and advice obtainable, even if this necessitates travel. This should not alienate your current health care team who know that the best road to health is the highest quality of treatment;

3) Avoid alternative treatments which are often costly rip-offs and can be dangerous at worst. Don't be afraid to mention these to your physician, who may have information about them or can access such information;

4) Enlist the support of family and friends;

5) Call upon whatever spirituality you have and ex-

pand it to envelope you with hope;

6) Attend to the quality of your life, avoid stress, hopelessness and isolation. If necessary make career changes and other situational changes to enhance and ease your life. Relaxation techniques and meditation are helpful stress reducers;

7) Make a conscious effort at self expression, particularly with your health care team, family and friends;

8) Keep a journal for both therapeutic benefit and for recording purposes. Remember that you are one of life's true heroes. Your courage is a tribute to carry with you as long as you survive.

BIBLIOGRAPHY

Achterberg, J., Matthews-Simonton, S., and Simonton, O.C. (1977), "Psychology of the Exceptional Cancer Patient: A description of Patients Who Outlive Predicted Life Expectancies," *Psychother: Theory, Res., Pract.*, 14, Pgs. 416-422.

Allen, A. (1981), "Psychosocial Factors in Cancer, *A F P*, 197-201.

Blandy, J.P., Oliver, R.T.D. and Hope-Stone, H.F. (1983), "A British Approach to the Management of Patients with Testicular Tumors" in J.P. Donohue (Ed.), *Testis Tumors*, Williams & Wilkins, Baltimore, Pgs. 207-223.

Bombeck, B. (1989), I Want to Grow Hair, I Want to Grow Up, I Want to Go to Boise, Harper & Row, New York.

Breitbart, W. (1987), "Suicide in Cancer Patients," *Oncology*, Vol. I, 49-54.

Bukberg, J., Penman, D. and Holland, J.C. (1984), "Depression in Hospitalized Cancer Patients," *Psychosom. Med.*, 46, Pgs. 199-212.

Cassileth, B.R., Lusk, E.J., Strouse, T.B., Miller, D.S., Brown, L.L., Cross, P.A. and Tenaglia, A.N. (1984), "Psychosocial status in cronic illness, a comparative analysis of sic diagnostic groups", *N. Engl. J. Med.*, 311, 506-511.

Cox, T. and Mackay, C. (1982), "Psychosocial factors and psycho-physiological mechanisms in the aetiology and development of cancers, *Soc. Sci. Med.*, 16, 381-396.

Dean, C. (1988), "The emotional impact of mastectomy", *Brit. J. Hosp. Med.*, 30-39.

de Haes, J.C. M. and van Knippenberg, F.C.E. (1985), "The quality of life of cancer patients: a review of the literature," *Soc. Sci. Med.*, 20, 809-817.

del Regato, J.A., Spjut, H.A. and Cox, J.D. (1985), *Ackerman and del Regato's Cancer, Diagnosis, Treat-*

ment and Prognosis, The C.V. Mosby Co., St. Louis, pp.705-721.

Derogatis, I.R., Morrow, G.R., Fetting, J., Penman, D., Piasetsky, S., Schmale, A.M., Henrichs, M. and Carnickle, C.L.M. (1983), "The prevalence of psychiatric disorders among cancer patients," *JAMA*, 249, 751-757.

Ell, K., Nishimoto, R., Morvay, T., Mantell, J. and Hamovitch, M. (1989). "A longitudinal analysis of psychological adaptation among survivors of cancer", *Cancer*, 63, 406-413 .

Evans, D.L., McCartney, C.F., Haggerty, J.J., Nemeroff, C.B., Golden, R.N., Simon, J.B., Quade, D., Holmes, V., Droba, M., Mason, G.A., Fowler, W.C. and Raft, D. (1988), "Treatment of depression in cancer patients is associated with better life adaptation: a pilot study", *Psychosom. Med.*, 50, 72-76.

Fiore, N. (1979), "Fighting cancer-one patient's perspective", *New Engl. J. Med.*, 300, 284-289.

Goldberg, R.J. (1983), "Psychiatric symptoms in cancer patients, is the cause organic or psychologic?", Postgrad. Med., 74, 263-273

Goldberg, R.J. and Cullen, L.O. (1985), "Factors important to psychosocial adjustment to cancer: a review of the evidence," *Soc. Sci. Med.* 20, 803-807.

Goodwin, J.S., Hunt, W.C., Key, C.R. and Samet, J.M. (1987), "The effect of marital status on stage, treatment and survival of cancer patients," *JAMA*, 258, 3125-3130.

Graves, P.L., Mead, L.A. and Pearson, T.A. (1986), "The Rorschach interaction scale as a potential predictor of cancer," *Psychosm. Med.*. 48, 549-563.

Green, R.L. (1987), "Psychosocial consequences of prostrate cancer - my father's illness and review of literature," *Psychosm. Med.*. 5, 315-327.

Greer, S., Morris, T, and Pettingdale, K.W. (1979), "Psychological response to breast cancer: effect on outcome," *Lancet* ii, 785-787.

Harris, A.E. (1988), "Physical disease and schizophrenia," *Schizo. Bul.* 14, 85-96.

Holland, J.C. and Massie, M.J. (1987), "Psychosocial aspects of cancer in the elderly," *Clin. Geri. Med.* 3, 533-539.

Ireland, J. (1987), *Life Wish*, Brown & Co., Boston.

Kaufman, M. (1989), "Cancer: facts vs. feelings," *Newsweek*, April 24.

Kriessel, H.T. (1987), "The psychosocial aspects of malignancy," Prim. Care. 14, 271- 280.

Krumm, S. (1982), "Psychological adaptation of the adult with cancer," *Nurs. Clin. N. Am.*, 17, 729-737.

Lansky, S.B., List, M.A. and Ritter-Sterr, C. (1986), "Psycho-social consequences of cancer," *Cancer*, 58, 529-533.

Lesk, S., (1988) "Psycho-oncology and psychoanalysis: some implications of modern research," presented before the 32nd annual meeting of the Amer. Acad. Psychoan., May 6.

Lickiss, J.N. (1980) "Psychosocial aspects of cancer," *Med. J. Aust.*, 1, 297-302.

Mack, R.M. (1884) "Lessons from living with cancer," *New Engl. J. Med.*, 311, 1640-1644.

Malec, J.F., Romsaas, E. and Trump, D. (1985) "Psychological and personality disturbance among patients with testicular cancer," *J. Psychosoc. Onc.* 3, 55-64.

McMahon, T.C. (1987) "Emotional distress and psychosocial adaptation in cancer patients," *Tex. Med.* 83, 44-47.

Northouse, L.L. and Swain, M.A. (1987) "Adjustment of patients and husbands to the initial impact of breast cancer," *Nurs. Res.*, 36, 221-225.

Peck, A. (1972) "Emotional reactions to having cancer," *Amer. J. Roentgenol. Radium Ther. Nucl. Med.* 114, 591-599.

Persky, V.W., Kempthorne-Rawson, J. and Shekelle, R.B. (1987) "Personality and risk of cancer: 20-year follow-up of the Western Electric study, " *Psychosom. Med.* 49, 435-449.

Plumb, M.M. and Holland, J. (1977) "Comparative studies of psychological function in patients with advanced cancer - 1. Self-reported depressive symptoms," *Psychosom. Med.* 39, 264-276.

Quigley, K.M. (1989) "The adult cancer survivor: psychosocial consequences of cure," *Sem. Onc. Nurs.* 5, 63-69.

Radner, G. (1989) *It's Always Something,* Simon and Schuster, New York.

Rainey, L.C. (1985) "Cancer counseling by telephone helpline: the UCLA psychosocial cancer counseling line," *Pub. Health Rep.* 100, 308-315.

Redd, W.H. and Jacobsen, P.B. (1988) "Emotions and cancer: new perspectives on an old question," Cancer 62, 1871-1879.

Rieker, P.P., Edbril, S.D. and Garnick, M.B. (1985) "Curative testis cancer therapy: psychosocial sequelae," J. Clin. Oncol. 3, 1117-1126.

Scherg, H. and Hum, S. (1987) "Psychosocial factors and disease bias in breast cancer patients," *Psychosom. Med.* 49, 302-312.

Schindehette, S. (1989) "Saturday night sweetheart," *People Weekly* June 5, 98-106

Schmale, A.H., Morrow, G.R., Schmitt, M.H., Adler, L.M., Enelow, A., Murawski, B.J. and Gates, C. (1983) "Well-being of cancer survivors," Psychosom. Med. 45, 163-169.

Searles, H.F. (1981) "Psychoanalytic therapy with cancer patients: some speculations," in J.G. Goldberg (ed.) *Psychotherapeutic treatment of cancer patients*, Free Press, New York, pp. 167-181.

Silberfarb, P.M., Maurer, L.H. and Crouthamel, C.S. (1980) "Psychosocial aspects of neoplastic disease: 1. functional status of breast cancer patients during different treatment regimens," *Am. J. Psychiat.* 137, 450-455.

Silverberg, E., Boring, C.C. and Squires, T.S. (1990) "Cancer Statistics , 1990" *Ca-a Canc. J. for Phys.* 40, 9-26.

Speigel, D., Bloom, J.R. and Yalom, I. (1981) "Group support for patients with metastatic cancer, a randomized prospective outcome study," *Arch. Gen. Psychiat.* 38, 527-533.

Stam, H.J., Butz, B.D. and Pittman, C.A. (1986) "Psychosocial problems and interventions in a referred sample of cancer patients," *Psychosom. Med.* 48, 539-548.

Wasserman, A.L., Thompson, E.I., Wilimas, J.A. and Fairclough, D.L. (1987) "The psychological status of survivors of childhood/adolescent Hodgkin's disease," *A.J.D.C.* 141, 626-631.

Wellisch, D.K. (1984) "Implementation of psychosocial services in managing emotional stress," *Cancer* 53, 828-832.

Worden, J.W. and Sobel, H.J. (1978) "Ego strength and psycho-social adaptation to cancer," *Psychosom. Med.* 40, 585-592.

Worden, J.W. and Weisman, A.D. (1980) "Do Cancer patients really want counseling?" *Gen. Hosp. Psychiat.* 2, 100-103

Zuromski, P. (1989) "Why do we get sick? A conversation with Dr. Bernie Siegel," Body, Mind and Spirit June 18-39

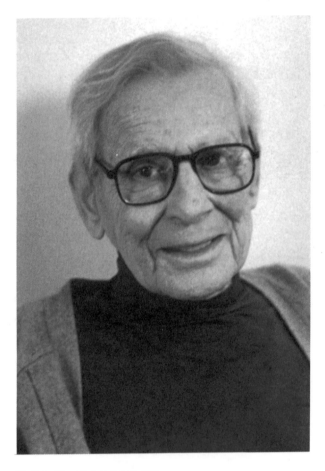

Photo courtesy of Leo H. Berman, M.D.

Stephen Fleck, M.D.

A LIFE TIME OF FACING DEATH

Stephen Fleck, M.D.

My first encounter with death occurred early, at least by today's standards when death in children and young adults has become rare in the developed world. When almost six, my three siblings and I were taken to a hospital - to say good-by to our father. It was maybe a week before he died of cancer. This was not, however, a very personal experience because I barely knew him and probably would never have recognized him in his emaciated state. He had been away in the German army for four years prior to his death. My only early recollection of him was seeing him once in his military uniform. I do not recall what, if anything, we were told about this death-bed visit. I only remember a week later that my mother screamed when she was informed that my father had died. We, at least my younger brother and I, were not included in whatever funeral there may have been. I only know that my father was buried in the Jewish cemetery in

Frankfurt, which my mother visited often, for many years. My mother never stopped mourning for him and had no social life beyond family gatherings. My father's death and the dire aftermath of World War I in Germany overshadowed our childhood.

Other deaths in the family occurred rather regularly during my childhood and adolescence. My paternal uncle died within five years of my father and an older maternal uncle died a year or two subsequent to that. The next relative to die was my maternal grandmother, with whom we had had almost daily contact. This death was especially sad for us but was mitigated by our employment of her long-time maid and cook. During my adolescence an aunt and a great aunt with whom I was close died. When I was nineteen I was employed by the hospital in which another maternal uncle was hospitalized and died from diabetes and kidney failure. His was the first death that I attended and witnessed.

My uncle's internist, a physician of international repute, tried to stem the rising uremia. He praised my uncle for every few drops of urine that my uncle produced. This scene appeared to me unreal and condescending, if not cruel, as no one knew how to reverse the deteriorating process. My uncle, the patient, was confused and was a non-participant in the decision process. For me the situation was both superfluous and undignified. I vowed never to impose this type of treatment upon a dying person.

My most disturbing exposure to death came during World War II, not during combat as an observer of combat-related death, but during the liberation of Buchenwald and Theresienstadt in the Russian zone. In both concentration camps people died from starvation even after they were "liberated." Witnessing these deaths emphasized one's complete helplessness. There were no facilities to treat, to nurture and perhaps to save these near-death concentration camp victims. Viewing death had been reduced for many to a routine experience.

While traversing much of Europe from Belgium and France to the former Czechoslovakia, death and destruction were a daily sight. Confronting death, even one's own, was necessitated by the still strafing Nazi planes.. After the Russians made contact with the U.S. Army, I probably came closer to death than I had earlier from enemy action. My ambulance driver and I, returning with a load of Theresienstadt inmates, were arrested by a Russian sergeant and his eager lieutenant who considered us spies. Luckily a Russian major who knew some German came along and decided that we shouldn't be killed but should return promptly to our lines. The Russians were prone to think that any stranger was an enemy or a spy who deserved to be killed; the U.S.' position as an "ally" did not completely reverse or even modify this perception. Despite the clear danger that the Russians had posed and conscious of the potentially fatal outcome, I experienced neither anxiety or excitement. I suspect internal denial was at work.

Soon after the episode with the Russian militia I was transported back to the States to be trained for the invasion of Japan. The atomic bomb effectively terminated this training. It wasn't until a year later with the publication of John Hersey's account in the *New Yorker* that the horror of the bombing and its ramifications became comprehensible.

Returning to civilian life ended any real danger to myself; I focused instead on the danger confronting the dying or the suicidal patient. This was an integral part of my psychiatric training, commenced after my return home. After 50 years of experience with psychiatric patients, I emphasize the hostile elements inherent in suicidal behavior i.e. approaching it from an interactional plane. I invariably correct the word "suicide" and term it "murder." Anecdotally speaking this seems to have a preventative impact.

During my residency I had occasion to discuss the issue of suicide with my retired father-in-law, who suffered from depression. He never did anything self-injurious and he died of natural causes some thirty years later. His wife died within a year. She was totally incapacitated by Alzheimer's Disease, perhaps one of the slowest deaths to impact on any family. This protracted illness emphasized our helplessness when faced with Alzheimer's or cancer. My father-in-law's good friend killed himself in a particularly gruesome way. This friend suffered from metastatic prostrate cancer. I again discussed the subject of reawakened suicidal intent with my father-in-law. When his wife, already well into Alzheimer pathology, took an overdose of barbiturates, he was offered options. He opted for "do everything you can" rather than opting for "no resuscitation".

Before my psychiatric residency and fellowship ended, I again confronted death. My sister died within six months of discovery of pulmonary metastasis from a breast cancer, which at the time of earlier surgical removal had been declared benign. The only treatment available at that time was radiation with which she had considerable exposure in her capacity as an x-ray technician. My sister did not believe - I think correctly - that this treatment would be effective. By this time she already had hepatic metastases.

Her physician kept her comfortable by not fighting or trying to delay the inevitable outcome. My sister and I were fortunate in having sympathetic internists and friends who felt comfortable with limiting care to palliation. She was 38 at this time, two years older than I. Ironically I was busy enjoying life with an 18 month old daughter. My son was born a month after my sister's death.

More recently a similar coincidence of a life beginning and another ending occurred. My wife died six years ago and our first grandson was born a week later. This most recent disaster was quite similar to my sister's in that my wife was discovered to have metastatic disease before the primary site (colon) and cause could be ascertained. Here again the question of debilitating treatment versus palliative measures to control pain and discomfort had to be made. We chose the latter approach. Again we fortunately had help from considerate and caring colleagues. My wife did not want to die but preferred a quiet passage without the unpleasant results of cancer therapies. She had witnessed these side effects during the cancer treatment and death of her sister eighteen months before.

As for myself, my wife's illness brought pain and difficulty in accepting the fatal inevitability of this disease. I believe, however, that when the body can no longer fight a disease, when there is no possibility of victory over the disease, that it is cruel and inhumane to delay the inevitable by prolonging life and its consequent misery. If the afflicted individual's decline is slow or care at home is not possible, hospice is available for appropriate care for both the patient and the family. (Nuland 1994)

Another "anticipated" death occurred some 12 years ago when a young nephew, barely 40, died from lung cancer. The first indication of cancer was a brain lesion which produced convulsions. His course was one of rapid descent, but there was an opportunity to discuss dying with him and custody arrangements for his son, the mother of whom was perceived to be untrustworthy. My contact with him during his last months were taken up not only with discussing death but appropriate arrangements to insure his son's welfare. He was consoled by these discussions, remained "outwardly peaceful" but continued to resent his fate and troubled a concerned staff with occasional angry outbursts. I felt and still feel, as do others, that we failed him despite trying to leave him peacefully. This was my first experience, aside from my "older" sister, with death in the younger generation. I believe that being able to anticipate death with the departing person seems to provide a consoling and grief-reducing opportunity.

In marked contrast sudden death is a different matter and I find it much harder to overcome. My first such experience was my mother's death, unexpected although she had suffered a coronary episode years prior to her death. I was in the military at that time and received a message that she had been hospitalized with pneumonia but was recovering well. Several days later I received a phone call that she had suffered a second and fatal heart attack. My fury at this time was boundless. I had requested and been denied emergency leave though I was not in a program where a few days absence would have affected the course of the war. I also experienced guilt. The much more disorganizing impact of a sudden unexpected death is noteworthy and I believe insufficiently recognized by most of us clinicians. An accidental or sudden death may not involve us to any great degree since we may not have seen the patient or his family prior to the death. My own reactions to sudden death in my family have alerted me to the hard-to-bear grief and sense of being wounded in sudden death situations.

Worse came more recently. My much beloved son-in-law turned up with a cystic kidney (he had only one having lost the other in an accident as a child) and predictably reached terminal kidney disease within a few years. He was on dialysis for some time which on the whole was successful within its limits. He ultimately after a long wait received a kidney transplant, which not only functioned effectively but altered his life back to that of a successful and gregarious young professional. Fourteen months after the transplant and without warning he suffered while asleep - a catastrophic myocardial infarction. He was found in the morning dead.

Mourning this young man's death has never ended. His death was reminiscent of my father's death at a similar age. My daughter confronted the situation and dealt with it far more effectively than my mother had. My daughter is now happily remarried.

An even worse disaster occurred some seven years ago when another nephew was murdered in his jewelry store. This young man had lived with us for several years during his early adolescence and was consequently even more like a child of ours than our son-in-law. Talking and thinking about him is hardly possible without feeling sad and angry. In both instances the notion that I should have passed away ahead of him has not dissipated.

Facing death has been far more prevalent and intense for me on a personal rather than on a professional basis. From the inception of my medical career, as a third and fourth year student and intern, I have not found it particularly difficult to talk with dying patients and their families. Occasions for this were, of course, much more common before I became a psychiatrist. In the latter role I have had only a few instances of having to deal with families after a suicide. My belief that suicide is a hostile act towards some significant other or others has not changed but it is an aspect that is difficult to deal with when you are expected to console families after such an event or even catastrophe. Guilt enters into the situation. Suicide is an unassailable criterion of failure, more so than death from an incurable disease.

If suicide occurs in an institutional setting, dealing and commiserating with its impact on staff is as important a task as meeting with the family and helping them to face the unalterable situation. Suicide is one fatal event which is preventable unlike death from cancer or complicated heart disease. I believe it is important to acknowledge such failure, even if it's not failure in the legal or technical sphere. What is most important in that situation is that the therapist or the institution has established constructive relationships with the patient's family or significant others. These preexisting relationships enhance the likelihood of being truly helpful to the survivors of suicide.

I have experienced more need to face the death of relatives and friends rather than patients. It has been my privilege to help colleagues deal with dying patients, because quite commonly physicians tend to avoid such patients. If they are the primary physician they may require assistance in coping with the situation rather than making a concerted effort to retreat from the patient that they can no longer help. This is particularly relevant with AIDS patients. One way a physician achieves distance is by prescribing heavy sedation or even antidepressants. A dying patient should be allowed to cry or be sad. I believe it is important to emphasize that dying patients never be left alone. If there is no professional attendant available, family members and/ or friends should be induced to remain with the dying person. It seems important to me that the dying should be accompanied to the end. In recent years I, as did my late wife, have attended a number of dying people as a friend or companion and not as their physician.

Returning to the issue of facing my own death, I am ready to die. I am not currently suffering from any fatal disease and have suffered from only two potentially fatal conditions. One was pneumonia during the flu epidemic in 1919. Although I was quite sick, I do not recall thinking or worrying about dying. Some seven or eight years ago I developed a violent gastroentero-colitis caused by nonsteroidal anti inflammatory medication for arthritis, emptying gastric and intestinal contents violently in both directions for several days. I perceived dehydration to be the only significant threat. My family, however, worried about me dying.

As previously stated I am ready to die but do not suffer from anything fatal, although plagued by arthritic pains and joint swellings controlled marginally by Bufferin. The aforementioned gastrointestinal problem has turned into chronic Crohn's Disease and colitis after resection of a constricted terminal ilium. Becoming anesthetized was so fast that I had no time to think or worry about anything. Some bleeding has kept me anemic for some time and probably will continue thus. All I can wish is that death will come suddenly - but not too suddenly for the children - without prolonged disability or confinement to bed.

Another non-fatal disability I have suffered is deafness. This, however, has been compensated for in the last two or three years by digital hearing aids which allow me to hear well in a quiet place, as well as to continue to enjoy music. This has provided a new lease on life. It is ironic that a professional whose work depends on listening should become deaf. Potential deafness became a real threat to my professional work until the newly developed hearing aids came to the rescue. Without the hearing aid my professional life would be severely curtailed if not rendered impossible. Other areas of my life would be subject to pervasive restrictions. These contingencies remain possibilities and could make me wish for a quick end. My life's work is mostly done. Regretfully I am not likely in the future to contribute or produce much of value to colleagues, family or friends.

BIBLIOGRAPHY

Gulati, S. (1988), "The Sound of a Thousand Cicadas", *Harvard Medical Alumni Bulletin* 73:29-33

Hersey, J. (August 31, 1946), "Hiroshima", *The New Yorker*

Nuland, S.B. (1994), *How We Die*, Alfred A. Knopf, New York, NY

INDEX

AUTHORS

AUTHORS

Listed Alphabetically

Earle L. Biassey, M.D.
Fellow, American Academy of Psychoanalysis

Diplomate of the American Board of Psychiatry and Neurology

Opal W. Broner, Ph.D.
Member, American Psychological Association

Edwin H. Church, M.D.
Fellow, American Academy of Psychoanalysis

Diplomate of the American Board of Psychiatry and
Neurology in Psychiatry

Leah Davidson, M.D.

Fellow, American Academy of Psychoanalysis

Fellow, American Psychiatric Association

Supervisor of Psychotherapy
White Institute, New York, NY

Training Analyst
The Institute of Health and Religion, New York,NY

Training and Supervising Analyst Emeritus
Long Island Institute of Psychoanalysis

Stephen Fleck, M.D.

Professor Emeritus, Psychiatry and Public Health
Yale University, New Haven, CT

Lester A. Gelb, M.D.

Fellow, American Academy of Psychoanalysis

Consultant Emeritus, Department of Psychiatry
Maimonides Medical Center, Brooklyn,NY

Associate Clinical Professor of Psychiatry
College of Medicine
Downstate Medical Center, Brooklyn, NY

Judita Hruza, M.D.

Diplomate of the American Board of Psychiatry and Neurology

Diplomate of the American Board of Pediatrics

Recipient of the Edward J. Hornick Memorial Award

Hae Ahm Kim, M.D.

Fellow, American Academy of Psychoanalysis

Diplomate of the American Board of Psychiatry and
Neurology in Psychiatry

Irvin A. Kraft, M.D.

Fellow, American Academy of Psychoanalysis

Emeritus Professor of Mental Health
University of Texas, School of Public Health
Houston, TX

Clinical Professor of Psychiatry
Baylor College of Medicine, Waco, TX

University of Texas School of Medicine, Houston, TX

University of Texas School of Medicine, Galveston, TX

Steven Lesk, M.D.

Fellow, American Academy of Psychoanalysis

Member, American Psychiatric Association

Senior Staff Psychiatrist
Anoka Metro Regional Treatment Center, Anoka, MN

George Nicklin, M.D.

Fellow, American Academy of Psychoanalysis

Fellow, American Psychiatric Association

Associate Clinical Professor of Psychiatry
N.Y.U. School of Medicine, New York, NY

Private Psychiatric Practice
Garden City, NY

Elizabeth Warner

Wife of Silas Warner, M.D.

Cornell University B.A. 1953

Silas Warner, M.D.

Fellow, American Academy of Psychoanalysis

Executive Committee
Philadelphia Academy of Psychoanalysis

Associate Clinical Professor of Psychiatry
University of Pennsylvania, Philadephia, PA

Psychiatric Consultant
Haverford College, Haverford, PA

Swarthmore College, Swarthmore, PA